Beating Melanoma

Beating Melanoma

A Five-Step Survival Guide

Steven Q. Wang, M.D.
Memorial Sloan-Kettering Cancer Center

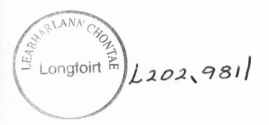

The Johns Hopkins University Press
Baltimore

Copyright © 2009, 2011 by Steven Q. Wang, M.D.
All rights reserved. Published 2011
Printed in the United States of America on acid-free paper
9 8 7 6 5 4 3 2 1

The Johns Hopkins University Press
2715 North Charles Street
Baltimore, Maryland 21218-4363
www.press.jhu.edu

An earlier version of this book was published on-line as
*Beating Melanoma—The Survival Manual:
A 5-Step Guide for Patients with Melanoma.*

Library of Congress Cataloging-in-Publication Data
Wang, Steven Q.
   Beating melanoma : a five-step survival guide / Steven Q. Wang.
      p. cm.
   "A Johns Hopkins Press health book."
   Includes index.
   ISBN-13: 978-0-8018-9889-1 (hardcover : alk. paper)
   ISBN-10: 0-8018-9889-7 (hardcover : alk. paper)
   ISBN-13: 978-0-8018-9890-7 (pbk. : alk. paper)
   ISBN-10: 0-8018-9890-0 (pbk. : alk. paper)
   1. Melanoma—Popular works. 2. Melanoma—Treatment—
Popular works. I. Title.
   RC280.M37W35 2011
   616.99'477—dc22   2010025897

A catalog record for this book is available from the British Library.

*Special discounts are available for bulk purchases of this book.
For more information, please contact Special Sales at
410-516-6936 or specialsales@press.jhu.edu.*

The Johns Hopkins University Press uses environmentally friendly
book materials, including recycled text paper that is composed of
at least 30 percent post-consumer waste, whenever possible. All of
our book papers are acid-free, and our jackets and covers are printed
on paper with recycled content.

The facing page constitutes an extension of this copyright page.

To my family, for their deep love and support

To Dr. Alfred W. Kopf, Dr. Harold S. Rabinovitz, Dr. David Polsky, Dr. Ashfaq Marghoob, Dr. Allan Halpern, Dr. Leonard H. Goldberg, and Dr. Kishwer Nehal for their continual guidance and support throughout my career

To Dr. Stephen Dusza, Dr. Richard Bezozo, Dr. Christopher Kruse, Dr. David Swanson, and my melanoma patients for their critical reviews of the manuscript

To Jacqueline Wehmueller and Anne Whitmore, my editors, for their professional excellence and for their many valuable suggestions

To Robert Tagliaferro, Melissa Delaney, Carolyn Corigliano, Jacklyn Carney, Brandee Hasko, and the rest of the dedicated dermatology staff at the Memorial Sloan-Kettering Cancer Center in Basking Ridge, New Jersey, who are committed to delivering the highest quality care to melanoma and nonmelanoma skin cancer patients every day

Contents

Color illustrations follow page 82.

Preface

The incidence of melanoma has risen dramatically over the past fifty years; more and more people are developing melanoma. It is estimated that in 2009 nearly 69,000 individuals were diagnosed with this skin cancer in the United States and nearly 8,650 people in this country died due to melanoma.

Melanoma can profoundly affect a person on many levels: physically, psychologically, emotionally, and economically. As a dermatologist and skin cancer specialist working at the Memorial Sloan-Kettering Cancer Center, I diagnose, treat, and care for many people with melanoma. I also care for people who are at high risk of developing melanoma. My work brings me into close contact with patients, who share their stories with me. These stories are moving, inspirational, touching, and, sometimes, sad. My interactions with patients have given me a deep appreciation for and understanding of the difficulties and challenges they face, especially in the beginning, when they are first diagnosed with melanoma.

When my patients are first diagnosed, they react with a range of emotions, from surprise, denial, frustration, and confusion to fear and even despair. However, this is not the time to panic. Denial is not an option. You need to take action and take action fast. Certainly, your physician will urge you to undergo treatments as soon as possible—and this urgency is necessary—but some of my patients say that they feel themselves losing control as soon as this process starts.

There is no doubt that you will go through an intense and stressful period from the time of diagnosis to the time when you complete treatment. I call this period the "mad rush." Many patients find this is a highly stressful time. They must quickly learn about the disease, seek experts near their home, and decide on treatment options. During treatment, many people feel that the process is chaotic and that they have lost control. Navigating the "mad rush" phase can be challenging, even for many health care professionals. That's why I wrote the first part of this book. Chapters 1 and 2 are designed to guide you through this phase.

Chapter 2 provides a step-by-step map through the "mad rush" phase. It will also help you become familiar with the vocabulary of melanoma, the relevant medical background information and basic treatment options, and information about survival outcomes which is tailored to different individuals' conditions and the stages of illnesses. Such knowledge can be extremely helpful when you are moving through the "mad rush" phase.

After successfully completing this phase, many people with melanoma feel a transient relief. At some point after treatment, however, most people who have had melanoma grapple with a fresh wave of questions and nagging concerns. They wonder if they will develop new melanoma or get other skin cancers. They wonder whether they need more treatments. They worry about whether their children and their siblings will also get skin cancer.

With each passing year after treatment, most melanoma survivors gain a deeper understanding of their disease and become more comfortable and reassured. They enter what I call the "marathon" phase. Information in the second part of this book, Chapters 3 and 4, addresses many of your lingering concerns and questions. These chapters will also help you to develop habits and practices that can prevent additional skin cancers.

I do not want to close this preface without saying a few words about cancer and attitudes toward cancer. In the United States and many other countries, the word "cancer" still carries frightful connotations. Many people consider cancer to be a death sentence. Luckily, this is far from the truth in developed countries. Modern medicine has made enormous strides in the diagnosis and treatment of cancer. Progress in computer technology, noninvasive imaging, gene therapy, and other new discoveries have changed the medical management of cancers. In fact, I would even go so far as to state that many types of cancer have been transformed into chronic, rather than terminal, diseases, much like high blood pressure and diabetes.

While melanoma is the most dangerous type of skin cancer, most people who are diagnosed early have excellent prognosis and survival outcomes. Treatment for early melanoma is straightforward and not complicated. Because of heightened public awareness of the signs of skin cancer and improved diagnostic techniques, more people today are diagnosed at an early stage. If you are diagnosed with melanoma at an early or intermediate stage of the disease, the disease can be treated relatively easily. And treating cancer early usually means you will have an excellent chance for survival.

How to Read This Book

If you have just been diagnosed with melanoma and have not yet received any treatment, you are in the "mad rush" phase. I recommend that you first read Chapter 1, which is a very brief introduction to melanoma, and then read Chapter 2, the step-by-step guide. Focus on understanding terminologies and the tasks ahead.

Chapters 1 and 2 will help you to work better with the team of physicians who will provide your treatment. You may want to read Chapter 2 more than once, for better understanding. When you have completed your treatment or you have more time, read the rest of the book. Be sure to use the "Beating Melanoma Checklist" in Chapter 5.

If you had a melanoma many years ago and have been treated, you are in the "marathon" phase. I recommend that you read Chapter 1 and then skip to Chapter 3 ("The 'Marathon' Phase: Surviving Melanoma") and Chapter 4 ("Networking: Finding and Sharing Information"). After you have read these chapters, you may find it helpful to read Chapter 2 and complete some of the tasks described there, such as obtaining copies of your old pathology reports. Please also review the appendixes, which illustrate different skin cancers.

Of course, you can read this book in the traditional fashion, from the beginning to the end. However, it is important to read it a few times, because stressful situations impair our ability to absorb new information.

There is a glossary at the back of the book that defines the technical terms used in this book. The index will help you find the pages where specific topics are discussed.

1. Introduction

You Have Melanoma. Now What?

Stephanie is a 31-year-old woman with light blonde hair, deep blue eyes, and fair skin. She grew up near the Atlantic Ocean, and each summer she would get sunburned. This is her third visit to our melanoma clinic, where she is due for her semiannual skin exam. Her melanoma was on her left leg. It was diagnosed and treated a few years ago, and she is doing well.

After asking Stephanie a few important questions about her overall health, I start my exam. As I proceed through my usual routine, Stephanie assures me that she is avoiding excessive sun exposure every day. I nod in approval. She is both nervous and happy when I tell her that I have not spotted any troublesome lesions on her upper body. As I move to examine her legs, I lean in for a closer look and feel the long scar on her left leg—the lasting remnant of her melanoma surgery—to check for any recurrence of the melanoma. Stephanie becomes silent and tense. Sensing her anxiety, I reassure her that everything looks good.

As I complete the exam, I again reassure her that she is doing very well. The scar on her left leg is well healed. I do not see any moles or spots that are worrisome. As she listens to me, her eyes and left hand wander to the scar on her left leg for a moment, and then she smiles in relief.

Stephanie's melanoma was diagnosed more than three years ago, in a fortuitous way. She was working as a pharmaceutical representative, visiting doctors in their offices to educate them about the latest drugs from her company. During a summer visit, a nurse pointed out a dark mole on her left leg and urged her to see a dermatologist about it. Heeding the warning, Stephanie made an appointment with her dermatologist, who shared the nurse's concern and removed the mole. One week later, Stephanie received a phone call. The dermatologist shared the bad news: "Stephanie, the mole we removed from your leg was a melanoma. It is a type of skin cancer that needs to be treated quickly."

Stephanie was stunned. Her dermatologist relayed information about her disease, but Stephanie did not remember any of it. When she hung up the phone, all she remembered was that melanoma is a type of skin cancer. Judging by the urgency and tone in her dermatologist's voice, she knew the situation was serious. She had made a note about her appointment the following week for surgery.

That night, she went home and told her husband about the diagnosis. They had heard of melanoma but did not know much about it. Soon, both Stephanie and her husband had a long list of questions, but it was too late at night to call her doctor. So they turned on the computer and started their own research on the Internet. Together they jumped from one site to the next and tried to grasp as much information as they could about melanoma. They encountered strange terms, such as "Breslow thickness," "sentinel lymph node biopsy," "isolated limb perfusion," and "interferon." They came across alarming warnings, such as: "Melanoma is the most dangerous type of skin cancer"; "One American dies from melanoma every hour"; "Lymph node dissection may be needed"; and "Patients need chemotherapy." The scariest statement they read was this one: "Currently, there is no cure for advanced stage melanoma."

Stephanie recalled the terrible experience of sitting beside her husband and sifting through those Internet sites. The information was scattered. The medical terminology confused her. The statistics and warnings terrified her. To make matters worse, some of the reputable sites repeated similar warnings. All she could think about was the impending big surgery, possible lymph node dissection, and possible chemotherapy. As she tucked in her baby girl that night, tears streamed down her face. She could not read or think about this anymore, and she could not wait for her next week's appointment. She decided that she would trust her dermatologist and hope for the best. Fortunately,

Stephanie was lucky. Her melanoma was at a very early stage. She only needed surgery to remove the tumor. There was no need for chemotherapy or other additional treatment. Stephanie was smart to take the advice of the nurse she encountered in the doctor's office.

Unfortunately, Stephanie's experience is all too common. Many melanoma patients spend anxious, tearful nights right after they hear the diagnosis. Being anxious is a normal feeling after hearing bad news. A person's temperament, life experiences, and support system all influence how they react to such news; not everyone reacts the same way or on the same schedule. Many people immediately seek additional information to help them cope, however—and that, too, is normal.

If you have received a diagnosis of melanoma, in addition to talking with your physicians, you may seek advice from friends or family members who have had melanomas. Some of these friends and family will be reliable sources of information, but keep in mind that much of what they can tell you about melanoma applies to *them*, not necessarily to you. Also, information that is passed on from a friend of a friend may get garbled in the relay and be wrong. You may want to speak directly with the person who had melanoma, if possible. Other people can tell you about some of the physicians in the area who provide expert care for people with melanoma, but again, for any number of reasons, one person's experience (favorable or not) with a specific health care provider may be different from another person's experience with that same health care provider.

Like Stephanie, many people seek answers through the Internet. The Internet is a convenient and familiar source of information for lots of people. (The informational Web sites that I recommend are listed at the end of Chapter 4.) Unfortunately, the information provided by many Web sites is fragmented, and *most of the information on Web sites is not relevant for most patients.* Reading a blog or other network posting that describes a person's experience is like talking to a stranger who has had melanoma. You will learn about that person's melanoma experience, but his experience is very likely to be different from yours. And you can't know whether the person writing on the Internet is a reliable source, or even whether that person truly had melanoma. Some of the information on the Internet is confusing, and confusing information can cause people to feel uncertain and fearful. Worst of all, some of the information on Web sites is incorrect.

Because melanoma should be treated quickly, urgency is needed in gathering information and deciding on the course of action. People worry about what to do during what I call the "mad rush" phase between initial diagnosis and beginning treatment. During this period, you will meet various specialists who will examine you, talk with you, help educate you, and work with you to come up with the best treatment plan. You will encounter unfamiliar words, statistics, and other data, and you may need to make serious decisions. Again, all this will happen quickly.

There is no way around the following fact: critical steps must be taken from the time of the initial diagnosis all the way to the treatment. My experience with patients has shown me that the best way to navigate through the "mad rush" phase is to have accurate, up-to-date information about melanoma and to have support from friends and family.

Newly diagnosed patients need reliable information *now*, and that is what this short book provides. In Chapter 2, I describe a five-step plan that will help you find information and make decisions during the "mad rush." The five steps are:

Step 1. Get the information
Step 2. Assess the reliability of the information
Step 3. Find the clinical experts in your area
Step 4. Understand your treatment options and the AJCC staging system
Step 5. Understand survival rate and prognosis

2. The Five-Step Plan

Navigating the "Mad Rush" Phase

Your physician has examined and biopsied the lesion of concern, the tissue sample has been sent to a medical laboratory for analysis —which confirmed the diagnosis of melanoma—and you have just been informed by your physician that you have melanoma. You are about to embark on the "mad rush" phase.

Step 1. Get the Information: The Pathology Report

The pathology report is an important medical document that includes valuable information about your diagnosis. The report is generated by a pathologist or a dermatopathologist (I'll explain the difference when we get to Step 2). The tissue sample that your dermatologist or family physician obtained from a skin biopsy is processed through a series of steps. First it is cut into very thin slices, 4 to 20 micrometers (μm) in thickness—which is thinner than the width of an average human hair. The slices are placed on a glass slide and stained with special dyes that help make the features of the tissue more visible and distinct.

A pathologist or a dermatopathologist examines the tissue sample through a microscope. The pathologist considers the appearance of the tissue, focusing on the shape and structure (called "morphology") of the cells and tissue within the specimen. Based on the microscopic observations about the tissue sample, the pathologist reaches a diagnosis, which is then recorded in the report.

The pathology report is crucial. The information in this report will help determine the management plan and plays a role in prognosis—in making a prediction about how likely it is that the patient will survive. The report is mailed, faxed, or delivered electronically to the physician who performed the biopsy, and the information is then conveyed to the patient by the physician or by someone else in the physician's office.

You need to have a copy of this report. Now for the easy part: to obtain a copy of the pathology report, just ask the dermatologist or the physician who performed the biopsy. By law, the physician must give a copy to you if you request it. You should then make a couple of photocopies of the report.

Why You Need a Copy of the Pathology Report

Once you are given the diagnosis of melanoma, you will embark on a long road of medical care: you will work with many physicians with different specialties. At each encounter with one of these specialists, the physician will need a set of basic information in order to plan treatment and decide on follow-up care. Almost all of them will want to read the information in your pathology report. When you arrive with this important document in hand, you will make the visit more productive and efficient. Without it, the specialist will not have the critical information and definitive evidence about the diagnosis to plan the appropriate treatment. Most physicians will not rely on a patient's words alone, because anyone can misremember information—especially information that is emotionally upsetting. So please remember to *bring a copy of the report with you each time you see a new physician.* If a copy of the report is not available at the time of your appointment, your treatment and your care may be delayed. I assure you: this type of delay can happen, and you want to avoid it.

You also need to read and understand the pathology report yourself. (This book will help you understand it.) You are about to begin working with medical professionals to tackle a serious disease, and you will need to know as much about this disease as possible so you can make sound decisions. Just as you gather information on automobiles or appliances before you decide which one to buy, you need to investigate and learn about your melanoma so you can make well-informed decisions. The saying "Knowledge is power" is based on experience.

Put a copy of the report in your permanent health file as well. In addition to needing a copy during the "mad rush" phase of dealing with melanoma, you will also need it during the marathon phase of dealing with melanoma, which may last many years and will involve continual follow-up with dermatologists and other physicians. During this phase, you may move to another geographic area, or you may change physicians. As you meet each new physician, he or she will want to know a great deal about your disease. Again, the physician will not want to trust your memory, and neither should you. It's human nature to forget crucial pieces of information contained in the pathology report.

Understanding the Report

When you first read the pathology report, you may not understand much of what it says, because pathology reports are written in medical jargon using technical terms. Let me assure you, though, that the information contained in the report is worth understanding and you can do it.

Here are a few basic things to do, when you get your report. Follow along in the sample pathology report (Figure 2.1) as you read this section. Different pathology labs use different report styles; your report may look different, and the crucial information may appear in different locations in your report, but the same elements should be there.

Basic Information

First, verify that your name and date of birth are accurate and that the correct date is given for when the biopsy specimen was submitted to the laboratory. Taking time to check these three pieces of information is necessary because you want to be sure that this report is for you and not for someone else.

The report will contain the name of and contact information for the physician who performed the biopsy. There should also be the name of and contact information for the pathologist or dermato-pathologist who made the diagnosis on this pathology report.

Diagnosis and Description

Each report contains the same necessary elements: the *diagnosis, microscopic description,* and *macroscopic description.* The microscopic description discusses the tissue features seen under the microscope. The macroscopic description provides details about the tissue specimen when it first arrived in the laboratory, before the tissue was processed in any way (that is, before it was cut and stained, as described above). You do not need to understand the macroscopic description, so we will focus on a few key points about the diagnosis and the microscopic description.

1. *Location of the biopsy.* Make sure the correct anatomic site is given. Check left versus right, to make sure the correct side of your body is identified. This is a common mistake in "path" reports. If the biopsy was on the leg, make sure the report states "leg" rather than some other part of the body.

2. *Diagnosis.* Make sure the diagnosis of melanoma or other diagnosis is clearly stated. If after reading the statements in the "diagnosis" section you do not see a diagnosis, be sure to ask your dermatologist for an explanation.

3. *Is it "in situ" only?* This is the next question to keep in mind when reading your pathology report. In the report, you may see the words "in situ." The term *in situ* means that the tumor has not penetrated beyond the epidermis (the outermost layer of the skin). If the pathology report states that the melanoma is an "in situ" lesion, then the treatment is very straightforward: the lesion can be simply removed. Chances for survival and cure are excellent with in situ tumors. If your melanoma is an in situ lesion, you can skip items 4 to 8 below, as this information will not be applicable to your case. You can move on to Step 2.

Figure 2.1 *(opposite)* Example of a pathology report.

```
Patient:                              Accession #:  509-4960
MRN:                                  Service:  Dermatology
Account #:                            Date of Procedure:  2/2/2009
DOB:          (Age:  67)  M           Date of Receipt:  2/2/2009
Physician:  Steven Q. Wang, M.D.      Date of Report:  2/10/2009 21:35
CC:
Patient Address:
```

Clinical Diagnosis & History:
Rule out melanoma.

Specimens Submitted:
1: SP: SKIN, LEFT BACK; EXCISION (mvm)

DIAGNOSIS:
1: SP: SKIN, LEFT BACK; EXCISION (mvm):
    Tumor Type:
        Malignant melanoma, in situ and invasive

Breslow thickness:
        0.2mm

Ulceration:
        Not identified

Mitotic index:
        $0/mm^2$

Clark level:
        II

Surgical Margins:
        Not involved
        The distance between in situ melanoma and the nearest
        peripheral margin is 2.0mm

Infiltrating lymphocytes:
        Non-brisk

Regression:
        Identified minor

Lymphovascular invasion:
        Not identified

Perineural Invasion:
        Not identified

Microscopic satellite:
        Not Applicable

Comment: THE MELANOMA APPEARS TO BE ARISING WITHIN A DYSPLASTIC
MELANOCYTIC NEVUS.

Gross Description:
1). The specimen is received in formalin, labeled "Left back
excision to rule out melanoma" and consists of an ellipse of
white tan unoriented skin, measuring 3.1 x 1.5 x 0.5 cm. Roughly
at the central skin surface, a hypopigmented area is identified,
measuring 1.1 x 0.8 cm and located 0.2 cm from the nearest margin.
The margins are inked black and serial sectioning reveals
homogeneous yellow tan lobulated adipose tissue. On cut section,
the lesion measures up to less than 0.1 cm in depth, and does not
appear to extend to the deep margin of excision. The specimen is
serially sectioned from tip to tip and entirely submitted.

Figure 2.2. Breslow thickness measurement. The depth is measured in millimeters from the very top of the epidermis to the deepest melanoma cells in the skin.

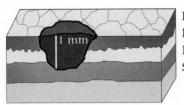

Epidermis
Papillary Dermis
Reticular Dermis
Subcutis (fat)

4. *Is it invasive? If yes, then what is the Breslow thickness?* In general, if the melanoma is not an in situ lesion, it is an invasive lesion. Invasive melanoma means the tumor has penetrated the epidermis—it has gone below the top layer of the skin. If the report clearly states "invasive melanoma," then look for the phrase "Breslow thickness."

The Breslow thickness is one of the most important pieces of information in the report. Breslow thickness measures the depth of penetration by the tumor cells. It is measured from the very top of the epidermis to the deepest melanoma cells in the skin tissue (see Figure 2.2). The unit of measurement is millimeters. If you have trouble finding this information, look for a number followed by the abbreviation "mm" (for example, 0.5 mm, 1.2 mm or 0.2 mm). Again: *Breslow thickness is one of the crucial pieces of information that will identify the stage of the disease, determine treatment options, and help predict survival rate. It is vital information.*

5. *Mitosis.* This term indicates cells undergoing division, splitting from one cell into two cells. Tumors grow by mitosis; as a tumor expands, the number of tumor cells increases. The pathologist can tell which cells are in the process of mitosis. The number of tumor cells undergoing mitosis reflects the activity of the tumor. In general, tumors with a high number of mitoses (cell divisions) are more aggressive, and therefore more worrisome. This is one of the important pieces of information needed to accurately identify the stage of melanoma if the lesion has a Breslow thickness of less than 1 millimeter (written "<1 mm").

Figure 2.3. Clark levels of measurement.

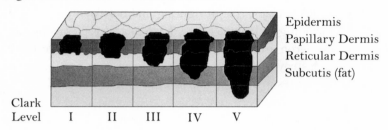

6. *Ulceration.* As the name suggests, ulceration indicates a loss of the intact skin overlying the tumor. Ulceration often indicates an advanced stage of disease and is another of the important pieces of information needed to accurately identify the stage of the disease.

7. *Clark level.* The Clark level is another way to describe the depth of melanoma invasion. Clark level is a five-level grading scale (see Figure 2.3).

- Level I describes tumor growth down to the junction between the epidermis (first layer of the skin) and the papillary dermis (top of second layer of the skin).
- Level II describes lesions that have penetrated the first layer of the skin but have invaded only the papillary dermis, a very superficial part of the dermis (second layer of the skin).
- Level III describes lesions that have extended to the border between the papillary (superficial) and the reticular (deep) layer of the dermis.
- Level IV describes lesions that have penetrated into the reticular (deep) layer of the dermis.
- Level V describes lesions that have extended into the subcutaneous layer, the fatty tissue layer of the skin.

Clark level is not as important in staging the disease as it once was, but many pathologists may still report this information. It is important not to confuse the Clark level with disease stage. The numerical designations for Clark level (I–V) mean something completely different from the numerical stage of the disease. For example, Clark level III does not mean stage III disease. Stages of disease will be discussed in Step 4.

8. *Lymphocytic infiltration.* Lymphocytes are the body's immune cells. They play a major role in fighting and destroying disease in the body, including melanoma cells. Melanoma therapies using vaccines or interferon aim to boost the ability of these cells to track, target, and destroy the melanoma cells. The presence of "brisk" or active lymphocytes in a melanoma is a good sign.

Pathology reports vary in the amount of detail they include. Most will contain the information described in items 1 through 5 above. For in situ melanoma, the information in numbers 4 to 8 above may not be included in the report, because it would not applicable.

Step 2. Assess the Reliability of the Information

Which Specialist Makes the Diagnosis?

At the beginning of this chapter I used the terms *pathologist* and *dermatopathologist.* Both refer to types of physicians who examine tissue under a microscope, render a diagnosis, and generate pathology reports. What are the differences between these specialists?

Pathologists are trained to examine tissue from all parts of the human body, such as the brain, muscle, colon, heart, and bone. By and large, most pathologists do not specialize in looking at skin tissues; that is, they do not exclusively examine skin tissue on a daily basis. In contrast, dermatopathologists are dermatologists or pathologists who have received additional training in examining skin specimens. They are focused on skin diseases. In general, dermatopathologists are more knowledgeable when it comes to skin disease. However, the important point is not whether a pathologist or a dermatopathologist reviewed the slides and made the diagnosis, but rather whether the physician who made the diagnosis is experienced and knowledgeable when it comes to melanoma.

Why Does It Matter Which Pathologist?

When it comes to melanoma, it is crucial to have an experienced and knowledgeable physician study the tissue under the microscope and make the final diagnosis. I learned this lesson very early on in my medical training and have seen it borne out many times since then, as the examples that follow will illustrate.

There are several reasons you should step back and assess the reliability of the diagnosis. First, there are skin lesions or tumors that can look like melanomas both clinically and under the microscope but are not melanoma. I have seen patients whose diagnosis of melanoma was changed to a severe dysplastic nevus (a type of atypical mole) after an experienced dermatopathologist or pathologist was asked to render a second opinion on a pathology slide. Another type of benign mole, called a Spitz nevus, can also mimic melanoma. I vividly remember a young woman who wept tears of relief after learning that she did not have a deeply invasive melanoma. Instead, she had a Spitz nevus. As a result of a change in the diagnosis made by a second, more experienced, dermatopathologist, she did not need to undergo a very large excision, sentinel lymph node biopsy, or other, more aggressive, treatments. (Sentinel node biopsy is explained later in this chapter.) A second, more knowledgeable, opinion helped her avoid extensive surgery and toxic systemic treatments and the problems associated with them—all of which would have been unnecessary for her.

Second, it is of the utmost importance to obtain an accurate Breslow thickness, measurement of the depth of melanoma cells in the skin. Breslow thickness dictates the treatment plan. Patients with thicker Breslow measurements need more aggressive treatment. The Breslow thickness is also used as an indicator for predicting survival. However, *measuring the deepest tumor cells in the skin tissue can be a challenge in certain cases.* As in many highly skilled tasks, experience and knowledge matter in taking these measurements. Inaccurate measurement of the tumor thickness can have dire consequences. Overestimation of the Breslow thickness can lead to an unnecessarily large surgery, longer surgical scars, and slower recovery time. Even worse, an overestimation of tumor thickness may lead to more invasive surgical procedures, such as a lymph node biopsy, or to unnecessary chemotherapy. On the other hand, underestimation of the Breslow thickness can lead to inadequate surgical intervention and inappropriate treatment, which have the potential for causing the melanoma to recur or spread.

The significance of expertise was illustrated in a clinical study conducted by a group of medical researchers from the Netherlands. The investigators submitted nearly two thousand lesion samples for a second opinion to the expert dermatopathologists and pathologists of the Dutch Melanoma Working Group Pathology Panel. The experts changed the diagnoses in 27 percent of the cases—more than one in every four. Thus, it matters greatly that you get an accurate diagnosis from a specialist experienced in diagnosing skin cancer based on biopsied tissue.

How to Verify the Accuracy of the Diagnosis

How can you assess the reliability of your diagnosis? The easiest approach is to talk to your dermatologist or the clinician who performed the biopsy of the skin lesion. *Ask whether he or she has confidence in the pathologist or dermatopathologist who read the slides.* Also, you can look at the pathology report. Usually at the end of the report, the pathologist or dermatopathologist will state if he or she is board certified in pathology or dermatopathology.

What to Do if You Are Not Satisfied with the Diagnosis

Sometimes the pathology report will not show a clear diagnosis. The pathologist or dermatopathologist may provide a microscopic description that is loaded with detail but does not state a diagnosis. This happens because in biology, as in nature in general, things are not always black and white—sometimes, they're gray. At times it is difficult to know whether a lesion is a melanoma or a severe atypical nevus, for example. But a pathology report without a clear diagnosis is troubling and doesn't provide the guidance your dermatologist needs to choose the best treatment. If the pathologist's report is unclear or is unsatisfactory to you in any way, you or your physician may wish to seek a second opinion; the same slides taken from the original biopsy can be reviewed by another, ideally more experienced, dermatopathologist. A second opinion does not mean a second sample of tissue must be taken. Just ask your physician, "Please have the slides reviewed by another dermatopathologist to

confirm the diagnosis." These are the words that many dermatologists use in talking to each other about difficult cases. If you
don't feel comfortable using this language, here is another way to
make the request: "Dr. Smith, I trust your judgment. Do you think
it may be a good idea to ask another dermatopathologist or pathologist who is experienced in melanoma to review the slides and
to confirm the diagnosis?" Remember, you want a board certified
and experienced dermatopathologist or pathologist to review your
slides.

If you and your physician decide to have the slides reviewed, it
is important to move quickly. The process usually takes four to ten
days and usually involves mailing slides from one lab to another.
The consulting dermatopathologist or pathologist will review the
slides and make his or her diagnosis. The results will be commu-
nicated to your physician through phone calls, e-mail, or fax. This
review and reporting of the opinion needs to be accomplished in a
speedy manner, so if you have doubts about the diagnosis, do not
delay discussing them with your physician.

When you receive the second diagnosis from your physician,
proceed again with Step 1: obtain a copy of the pathology report
and examine the information on it. Now you will have two reports
in hand. You can compare them. Your dermatologist should explain the results to you in detail, but you can familiarize yourself
with the report. In checking the second pathology report, here are
few important steps:

- Again confirm that the report is for you, not for someone
  else. Check the *pathology accession number* in both reports. The
  accession numbers on both reports should be identical. This
  means that the new dermatopathologist has looked at the
  same specimen.
- Make sure that the report is for a sample from the correct
  anatomical site. For example, if you had three biopsies but
  only the lesion on the left leg was in question, make sure the
  second report is generated for the left leg and not for the
  other lesions. Although mistakes are rare, they *can* happen.
  I have seen it.

- If the diagnosis is melanoma, is it described as invasive or in situ? If invasive, compare the Breslow thickness measurement with that in the first report, if it had one.

If the two sets of independent reviews of your slides come to the same conclusion, you will have assurance of the accuracy and reliability of your diagnosis.

What to Do if the Reports Conflict

Once in a while, two pathologists examining the same slides will have different findings and offer different diagnoses. If you obtain a second pathology report that differs from the first report, you can have a third dermatopathologist or pathologist review the slides.

Step 3. Find the Clinical Experts in Your Area

Let's assume that you have taken the first two steps. First, you have the pathology report in hand and are able to understand the key information. Second, you and your doctor are satisfied with the accuracy of the diagnosis. (If you have not carried out the first two steps, keep reading, anyway. You can always come back and review this section again after you obtain the pathology report.)

At this point, you have not had treatment for your cancer. The initial skin biopsy was done only to sample the skin tissue and make a diagnosis. During the biopsy, the physician removes a portion of or the entire lesion. Your physician may simply shave the worrisome mole with a razor blade–like instrument. In this procedure, no sutures (stitches) are needed to close the wound. Your physician may do a "punch biopsy": using a pencil-shaped device, the lesion is "punched," or cut out. Sutures are usually used to close the wound after a punch biopsy. Or, your physician may perform an "excisional biopsy." This method is more involved and is used to biopsy larger lesions. An elliptical-shaped section of skin is removed with a scalpel, a surgical blade. The wound is closed (sutured) in a linear fashion. In many cases, the surgical techniques and instruments used in excisional biopsy and a "definitive excision" (complete removal) of the melanoma are the same. The biopsy is done to obtain a sample of tissue; the definitive excision is done to remove all cancerous tissue. Patients sometimes get confused between the procedures for a biopsy and for definitive treatment, and the confusion is understandable.

As you embark on the treatment phase, Step 3—finding the clinical experts in your geographic area—will be very important. Treatment options vary depending on many factors. These include Breslow thickness, mitosis, Clark level, ulceration, anatomical location, your age and health, and most importantly, the stage of disease (described under Step 4). The physician or team of physicians (which I will refer to as *clinical experts*) who are involved in your care will play a crucial role in the success or failure of your outcome. Their expertise, judgment and knowledge about melanoma and treatment matter! Inadequate or ineffective treatment can potentially lead to recurrence or metastasis of the disease, which can be fatal. In contrast, overly aggressive treatment can lead to unnecessary physical suffering and psychological trauma. This point is illustrated by the following two stories. (Stacy is currently my patient. Helen's story was shared by an oncologist who is in charge of various clinical trials for patients with advanced stages of melanoma.)

Stacy's and Helen's Stories

It was summer when I first met Stacy, a 32-year-old woman and a melanoma survivor. Her melanoma (Breslow thickness 0.4 mm), located on her left knee, had been diagnosed and treated more than one year before I met her. Her treatment course was long and arduous, lasting nearly the full year. After the initial biopsy, she quickly underwent surgery to remove the tumor and a standard margin of normal tissue. Her recovery was complicated by poor wound healing. The scar spread open and took a month and a half to heal. In addition, she had a sentinel lymph node biopsy (this procedure is discussed under Step 4) in the left side of her groin. After the surgery, the surgeon referred her for a chest CT scan. The CT scan showed a few questionable spots in one of her lungs. Stacy informed her doctor that she was a smoker, and her doctor recommended that she have a total body PET scan to further examine those spots and check for other irregularities. The PET scan showed that her lung was normal, but it indicated that there was a suspicious spot on her right ankle. She then proceeded with an MRI and a bone scan to look for the "hot" spot on her right ankle. Neither of these imaging studies was definitive. To finalize the work-up, she had a bone biopsy on the right ankle, the results of which were benign (normal). This ordeal took nine months. When Stacy shared this story with me, tears trickled down her face. She recalled how concerned she was going from one doctor to the next and having one test after another.

After the diagnosis and treatment of her melanoma, Stacy was told to have routine follow-ups with her local dermatologist. She had many moles. On each visit, her dermatologist found some moles that were worrisome. On virtually every visit, 1 to 3 moles were removed. All of these subsequent biopsies were benign; those moles were not melanomas. By the time I met Stacy, she had at least 15 small scars scattered over her body. Afraid of being "skinned alive," she came to our dermatology clinic at a cancer center for a second opinion regarding ongoing follow-up.

Helen was a woman in her early thirties who lived in England. Her melanoma was diagnosed at a very late stage. The melanoma cells had spread to her lungs and liver. She hoped to come to the United States to find a cure. Because of Helen's poor health, her doctors in England advised her not to make a trans-Atlantic journey. Ignoring her doctors' warnings, she came to a specialty cancer institute in the United States. Repeat clinical work-ups, involving blood tests and various imaging studies, confirmed that her melanoma was advanced. Her PET scan showed multiple tumors in her lungs and liver.

Helen immediately was started on a cocktail of systemic drugs that targeted the melanoma cells, boosted her body's immune system, and slowed the growth of new blood vessels that would feed the tumors. Within three months, Helen's disease had melted away. Her repeat PET scan showed clearance of the prior "hot" nodules in the liver and lungs. Her success story was nothing short of a miracle. The cocktail of treatments fought off the tumors.

Both of these women's stories are memorable. There is a stark contrast in their care. Stacy was subjected to overaggressive examination. She had a very early disease. Her melanoma was only 0.4 mm in Breslow thickness; she did not need a sentinel lymph node biopsy. The current recommendation is that sentinel lymph node biopsy should be done if the melanoma has a Breslow thickness greater than 1 mm, although some studies have shown that sentinel lymph node biopsies should be considered for certain patients with melanomas greater than 0.75 mm. In either case, Stacy did not need a lymph node biopsy. It is hard to argue whether the imaging studies were justified. However, one outcome is certain. These studies led to an unnecessary bone biopsy, an invasive procedure that left Stacy with recurring pain in her ankle. It is extremely unlikely that an early melanoma on one leg would jump and spread to the ankle on the other leg. Moreover, imagine the fear, the sleepless nights, and the anxiety that she and her husband endured in that year. Lastly, her dermatologist, in an effort to detect new melanomas, started biopsying many benign moles and left her with many unnecessary scars on her body. In contrast, Helen was on her death bed before being rescued by a team of specialists focused on melanoma care. Defying her own doctors' advice in England, she sought out the most expert care and became disease free.

The point of sharing both stories is neither to vilify nor to glorify any of the doctors involved. The message is simply this: *You need a qualified and expert team of physicians to take care of you!* In Stacy's case, what should have been a straightforward treatment for an early melanoma turned into a year of continual tests, complications, and possibly some unnecessary procedures. In Helen's case, a young woman with an advanced stage of disease found hope when her original doctors had given up on her. Again, *the key to successful treatment rests on finding clinical specialists,* preferably in your local area but if necessary elsewhere, who have the relevant expertise. *When handled by inexperienced physicians, patients with any stage of disease may have poor outcomes.*

How to Find Experts Near Your Home

To identify clinical specialists with expertise in melanoma, you will need to do some research. Here is some guidance in how to go about it.

First, specialists working in major academic medical centers or cancer centers tend to have more experience in dealing with melanoma, especially with advanced stages of this cancer. I would advise people with aggressive or late stage disease to seek care at a facility designated by the National Cancer Center as a comprehensive cancer center. Most physicians in these types of institutions have more experience and support in treating people with melanoma. Often, the care provided in these institutions is orchestrated by a team of specialists, including dermatologists, medical oncologists, surgical oncologists, radiation oncologists, dermatopathologists, and plastic surgeons, as well as nurses, psychologists, and social workers who provide supportive and practical care. Furthermore, some of these specialists have unique research interests in caring for melanoma patients and therefore they keep up to date with the latest research or clinical evidence and factor in the latest information when deciding on what care is best for each patient.

This is not to say that physicians who work outside of major hospitals or cancer centers are not able to care for melanoma patients. In fact, many melanoma survivors are treated and cured by physicians who are not working in one of these centers. Some of these physicians may even have spent years working in academic institutions or cancer centers before leaving those institutions for private practice or other medical settings.

I will explain the different stages of disease in detail in Step 4, but I want to say here that people who have intermediate or late stage disease should consider receiving their care in major institutions that have strong teams of melanoma experts.

Second, on your home or library computer conduct a search on PubMed (http://www.ncbi.nlm.nih.gov/sites/entrez/) or on Google Scholar. Both sites are excellent resources for the latest clinical and basic science research. PubMed provides an index of scientific articles. Simply type "melanoma" or "melanoma treatment" into the search window and you will see a long list of published articles. Now, look at who wrote these articles. Many of these authors have strong interests in the diagnosis and treatment of melanomas. Many are recognized as the experts in the field. Look at their institutional affiliations and you will be able to tell where they work.

Third, ask your dermatologist where you can receive the best treatment. Dermatologists are usually the practitioners who biopsy lesions and diagnose melanoma. For early stage disease, many dermatologists will themselves perform the necessary surgical procedures to remove the melanomas. However, some may refer you to other specialists, such as plastic surgeons or oncologic (tumor) surgeons and oncologists (cancer doctors) for consultation and treatment. You may like and trust your dermatologist, but how do you know if these other physicians are qualified? The quickest way to begin assessing the capability of those other physicians is to ask your dermatologist about them. Ask: "How good is the surgeon or the oncologist? How long have you worked with him or her?" Better yet, ask, "Would you refer your own mother to see this specialist?" The last question is a litmus test. It is a good sign if the dermatologist looks you straight in the eyes and tells you, "Yes, I would." In general, good physicians work with good physicians. Long periods of collaboration among different specialists reflect a sense of trust and approval for each others' work. No good physician will continue to refer his or her own patients to an unqualified physician.

Fourth, ask around. If you have friends or family members who had melanomas, call them. Ask about their experience. Get the name and contact information of their doctors. Word of mouth is often helpful.

Finally, if you have melanoma, you need to see a physician who is devoted to and interested in caring for people who have melanoma. Look for the doctor's practice or institutional Web site on the Internet. Many medical offices and medical institutions have informative Web sites detailing the credentials, knowledge, experience, and specific services of the physicians in those institutions or offices. You can learn a great deal by visiting their Web sites. Focus on the overall appearance and content of the site. You can make some educated guesses about whether a particular doctor is suitable for you. For instance, if you plan to see a dermatologist for melanoma follow-up, but on that dermatologist's Web site the only information you see is related to cosmetic services, such as Botox and laser treatment, and there is no mention of skin cancer treatment, this dermatologist is probably not the ideal person to care for your melanoma.

A number of independent Web sites have been created to rank doctors. In my opinion, these sites do not provide an objective measurement for assessing a physician. In most cases, the comments posted on these sites heavily focus on a physician's bedside manner. These sites also tend to be biased, since comments come from patients who are either extremely pleased or extremely displeased with the doctor.

What to Do if You Cannot Find Experts Near Your Home

If you live in an area where there are no melanoma experts, depending on the stage of the melanoma, you may wish to consider seeking care or a consultation in another location, as Helen did. If you live in the United States, you probably do not need to leave the country. The United States has some of the best medical institutions in the world. If you are able to travel, you can seek a consultation at one of these institutions, even if you don't live nearby. Experts in the institution can make recommendations for a treatment plan, and then your local doctors can deliver or perform the treatment recommended by these experts.

If you wish to explore the credentials of a specific physician or search for a board certified physician in an academic medical center or a cancer treatment center, you might find the following Web sites helpful.

For physicians' qualifications, check
- The American Board of Medical Specialties at www.abms.org
- The American Medical Association's AMA Doctor Finder at www.ama-assn.org/aps/amahg.htm

For hospitals, consult
- US News Hospital Ranking for Treating Cancer at health.usnews.com/best-hospitals/rankings/cancer
- National Cancer Institute Designated Cancer Centers at http://cancercenters.cancer.gov/cancer_centers/cancer-centers-names.html

Step 4. Understand Your Treatment Options and the AJCC Staging System

In Step 4 we will focus on the American Joint Committee on Cancer (AJCC) staging system, which was created to classify cancer according to the severity of the disease. This is called "staging the disease," a step that helps to determine the appropriate treatment. The system is also used to predict survival outcome. Understanding the technical information in this section of the book will provide you a solid foundation for understanding what is happening and knowledge that will help you discuss your treatment plan with your doctor. After reading this section, your interaction with your physician will be more productive and you will feel more in control.

Please note that understanding the staging system only provides you with the framework for more-useful interactions with your doctors. The first three steps, and especially finding the right experts, will influence the overall outcome of your care. Ultimately, it is your doctors who will guide and treat you.

What Is the AJCC Staging System?

The American Joint Committee on Cancer is a scientific group whose work is focused on cancer. The AJCC staging system is widely used as a road map by clinicians who are making decisions about the treatment of cancer patients. Patients with early stage disease need less aggressive treatment and have better survival outcomes. In contrast, patients with advanced disease need more aggressive treatment and tend to have more serious outcomes.

The latest version of the AJCC staging system for melanoma was published in 2009. The scientific committee reviewed a comprehensive database of prognostic (survival) factors based on reviewing data about 38,918 patients from 17 cancer centers and organizations. The committee wanted the staging system to be practical and applicable to the needs of various medical specialties. They also wanted the staging criteria to reflect the biology of melanoma. The criteria are based on medical and scientific evidence, and they reflect rigorous statistical analyses.

Interpreting the AJCC Staging System

Identifying the stage of cancer using the AJCC staging system depends on a number of important factors. These include:

Breslow thickness
mitosis
ulceration
lymph node involvement
other organ involvement

As noted in the discussion of Step 1, information about the Breslow thickness, mitotic rate, and ulceration can be found in the pathology report, based on the initial biopsy. To assess whether the melanoma has spread to any lymph nodes or other organs, additional examinations and tests, such as lymph node biopsy, blood work, or imaging studies, must be performed.

The AJCC staging system is based on the TNM classification, a reference to three of the criteria the system considers: the T stands for the tumor status; the N stands for lymph node involvement; and the M stands for metastasis of the disease, spread to other skin sites or to lungs or other visceral organs, such as the brain or liver. Table 2.1 explains the designations (for example, T2b) in the TNM classification for melanoma. The T component of the TNM classification is based on the information from the pathology report (such as Breslow thickness, mitotic rate, and ulceration). Table 2.2 shows how the TNM designations are combined to produce the AJCC staging system designations. Both tables can serve as a guide to the

Table 2.1 TNM Classification System for Melanoma

Tumor (T)	Thickness	Ulceration/Mitosis Status
in situ	NA	Not Applicable
T1	≤1 mm	a: Without ulceration and mitosis <1/mm^2 b: With ulceration or mitosis ≥1/mm^2
T2	1.01–2.00 mm	a: Without ulceration b: With ulceration
T3	2.01–4.00 mm	a: Without ulceration b: With ulceration
T4	> 4.0 mm	a: Without ulceration b: With ulceration

Lymph Nodes (N)	No. of Metastatic Nodes	Nodal Metastatic Burden
N0	0	Not Applicable
N1	1	a: Micrometastasis (diagnosed by sentinel lymph node biopsy) b: Macrometastasis (clinically detectable nodal metastases)
N2	2–3	a: Micrometastasis (diagnosed by sentinel lymph node biopsy) b: Macrometastasis (clinically detectable nodal metastases) c: In transit metastases/satellites without metastatic nodes
N3	4+ metastatic nodes, or in transit metastases/satellites with metastatic nodes	

Metastases (M)	Site	Serum Lactate Dehydrogenase
M0	No distant metastases	Not Applicable
M1a	Distant skin, subcutaneous, or nodal metastases	Normal
M1b	Lung metastases	Normal
M1c	All other visceral metastases	Normal
M1c	Any distant metastases	Elevated

Table 2.2 Summary of the American Joint Committee on Cancer (AJCC) Staging System

Stages	Tumor (T)	Nodes (N)	Metastases (M)
O	T in situ	N 0	M 0
IA	T 1a	N 0	M 0
IB	T 1b	N 0	M 0
	T 2a	N 0	M 0
IIA	T 2b	N 0	M 0
	T 3a	N 0	M 0
IIB	T 3b	N 0	M 0
	T 4a	N 0	M 0
IIC	T 4b	N 0	M 0
IIIA	T 1–4a	N 1a	M 0
	T 1–4a	N 2a	M 0
IIIB	T 1–4b	N 1a	M 0
	T 1–4b	N 2a	M 0
	T 1–4a	N 1b	M 0
	T 1–4a	N 2b	M 0
	T 1–4a	N 2c	M 0
IIIC	T 1–4b	N 1b	M 0
	T 1–4b	N 2b	M 0
	T 1–4b	N 2c	M 0
	Any T	N 3	M 0
IV	Any T	Any N	M 1

detailed explanation that follows. The AJCC staging system is more clinically relevant, because this is the information that determines the appropriate treatment and predicts survival outcomes.

To use the AJCC system, you need to first figure out your TNM status. As mentioned earlier, with the information on your pathology report, you can figure out the T component of the TNM status. For most early melanomas, the N and M will be zero, because the melanoma has not spread to the lymph nodes or other organs in the body. If you have any doubt about the N and M status, consult your physician. When you know your TNM status, then go to Table 2.2 and find your AJCC stage. Again, this information is provided only to serve as an educational guide. *You must discuss your medical condition and TNM classification and AJCC stage with your physician.*

AJCC Stages

Stage 0. A patient with stage 0 (zero) melanoma has in situ melanoma. In this stage, the melanoma has not penetrated beyond the epidermis (the top layer of the skin). Patients with this stage of melanoma have excellent survival outcomes. The melanoma can be treated with relative ease.

Stage IA. A patient with stage IA melanoma has a lesion with a Breslow thickness less than or equal to 1 mm. There is no ulceration in the tissue specimen, and there is less than 1 mitosis per square millimeter ($<1/\text{mm}^2$). Lastly, there is no evidence of lymph node involvement or other organ involvement. Patients with this stage of melanoma have excellent survival outcomes. The melanoma can be treated with relative ease.

Stage IB. A patient with stage IB melanoma may have one of two sets of melanoma features. Patients may have lesions with Breslow thickness less than or equal to 1 mm in which ulceration is present or the mitotic rate is $\geq 1/\text{mm}^2$, or patients may have lesions with Breslow thickness from 1.01 to 2 mm without ulceration. For both groups, there is no involvement of lymph nodes or other organs. Patients with this stage of melanoma have excellent survival outcomes. The melanoma can be treated with relative ease.

Stage IIA. A patient with stage IIA melanoma has one of two sets of melanoma features. Patients may have lesions with Breslow thickness from 1.01 to 2 mm with ulceration or lesions with Breslow thickness from 2.01 to 4 mm without ulceration. For both groups, the lymph nodes and other organs are not involved.

Stage IIB. A patient with stage IIB has one of two sets of melanoma features. Patients may have lesions with Breslow thickness from 2.01 to 4 mm with ulceration or lesions with Breslow thickness greater than 4 mm without ulceration. For stage IIB patients, the lymph nodes and other organs are not involved.

Stage IIC. A patient with stage IIC melanoma has a lesion with Breslow thickness greater than 4 mm in which ulceration is present. Lymph nodes and other organs are not involved.

Stage IIIA. A patient with stage IIIA melanoma has micrometastases of melanoma present in one, two, or three lymph nodes. *Micro*metastases in the affected lymph nodes cannot be palpated (felt with the hand) during a physical exam. Instead, the presence of melanoma cells in the nodes is detected by biopsying the lymph nodes. In this stage, ulceration is not present. In classifying stage III disease, the Breslow thickness does not play any role.

Stage IIIB. A patient with stage IIIB melanoma has melanoma cells in lymph nodes. There are two subgroups of stage IIIB. In the first group, patients have melanomas with ulceration, and there are micrometastases in one, two, or three lymph nodes. (As in stage IIIA, the presence of *micro*metastases cannot be felt during a physical exam but is detected by biopsying the lymph nodes.) In the second group, patients have melanomas without ulceration and there are *macro*metastases in one, two, or three lymph nodes. When *macro*metastases are present, lymph nodes *can* be palpated (felt) by the physician doing a physical examination of the patient. (There is more information about micrometastases and macrometastases later in this chapter.)

Stage IIIC. Patients with stage IIIC melanoma fall into two subgroups. In the first group are patients who have melanomas with ulceration and in whom there are macrometastases in one, two, or three lymph nodes. (Again, when macrometastases are present, the affected lymph nodes can be palpated or felt during a physical exam.) In the second group are patients with at least four affected lymph nodes, regardless of whether they are micrometastases or macrometastases.

Stage IV. The presence of "distant" metastatic disease elsewhere in the skin or in the lungs or other organs defines this stage. There are three subcategories (see Table 2.1). In the first subcategory are patients with only distant skin involvement, not other organs. In the second subcategory are patients with melanomas in at least one lung. In the third subcategory are patients with melanomas in organs other than skin and lungs, such as the brain, liver, and other visceral organs. For this stage, the Breslow thickness, Clark level, and ulceration do not play any role.

The intricacies of the staging system are extremely useful for physicians making decisions about treating patients and advising patients about their prognosis. The AJCC stages are based on data from real patients, and the distinctions among the categories reflect the survival outcomes in the treatment of melanoma.

How Does Your Doctor Identify the Stage of Your Disease?

As noted above, the AJCC staging system is based on the TNM classification, which is based on the Breslow thickness, mitosis, ulceration, lymph node status, and distant organ involvement. From the pathology report alone, your doctor can obtain the first three pieces of information: Breslow thickness, mitosis, and ulceration.

Patients with deep melanomas, as measured by Breslow thickness, tend to have or to develop advanced stages of the disease. The presence of ulceration increases the stage of the disease. If a patient has a melanoma with Breslow thickness of 1.5 mm without ulceration, he has stage IB disease. A patient who has a melanoma with the same Breslow thickness (1.5 mm) and ulceration has stage IIA disease. The presence of mitosis is important for melanoma with a Breslow thickness of less than 1 mm.

Lymph node involvement ("positive" lymph nodes—the presence of melanoma cells in lymph nodes) means the patient has stage III disease. Other organ involvement means the patient has stage IV disease. Neither the lymph node status nor other organ involvement is found on the pathology report from the original skin biopsy. The pathology report does not say whether the patient has any lymph nodes or distant organs involved with the melanoma, because skin biopsy does not provide any information about lymph nodes or other organs. Your doctor needs to perform additional examinations and tests to check the lymph nodes and other organs for metastases.

The next obvious questions are: *How does your doctor find out about the lymph node status?* and *How does your doctor find out whether there is involvement of other organs?* These questions (and others) are considered below.

How Does Your Doctor Check for Lymph Node Involvement?

To determine whether melanoma cells have spread from the primary site, in your skin, into the lymph nodes, your physician begins by feeling (palpating) the groin, armpits, and around the neck. Melanomas on the legs travel through the lymphatic channels and spread into the lymph nodes in the groin area. Melanomas on the arms tend to spread to lymph nodes in the armpits. Those on the trunk tend to spread to the armpits or groin nodes. And melanomas on the face, head, and neck travel to the lymph nodes around the neck. Once the cancer cells have spread to the lymph nodes, they can more easily travel on to other organs, because the lymphatic system runs throughout the body. If large lymph nodes can be felt in the groin, armpits, or neck and the presence of melanoma cells in the lymph nodes is confirmed by biopsy, this is referred to as *macrometastases* involvement.

For example, if a patient had an ulcerated melanoma on the left leg and a large lymph node in the left groin was palpable (able to be detected by hand), the patient would be suspected of having macrometastases. If subsequent biopsy of the lymph node confirmed the presence of melanoma cells, the patient's disease would be classified as stage IIIC disease. (This is stage IIIC because the melanoma is ulcerated [$T = 1–4b$] and has macrometasases [$N1b$].) It is important to note that many healthy individuals have small (3 mm to 4 mm in size), round and movable lymph nodes in the groin area. Usually, these small lymph nodes are found on both sides of the groin, not just on one side. *A person who has palpable lymph nodes does not necessarily have disease in the lymph nodes.* There are benign conditions that can explain the presence of palpable lymph nodes, as well as circumstances such as current or previous infections. To confirm the status of lymph node involvement, ultrasound or other studies or lymph node biopsies are needed.

What will happen if the physician does not find palpable lymph nodes when examining a person with melanoma? The physician may or may not order sentinel lymph node biopsy (described below) to check for the presence of micrometastases. By definition, *micro*metastases cannot be detected in a physical exam. With micrometastases, the presence of melanoma cells in lymph nodes can only be detected when these lymph nodes are biopsied and the tissue is examined under a microscope.

What Is a Sentinel Node Biopsy and How Does Your Physician Decide whether You Need One?

The sentinel node is the first lymph node that malignant tumor cells reach when cancer spreads from the original site. To determine which is the sentinel lymph node and perform a biopsy, the surgeon injects a small amount of blue dye mixed and tagged with a radioactive substance at the site of the melanoma, such as the leg or arm. The radioactive dye is used to trace the flow of lymph from the tumor to one of the lymph basins (the neck, groin, or armpit, depending on the site of the initial tumor, as described above). After making an incision in the lymph node region (the neck, groin, or armpit), the surgeon looks for lymph nodes with blue color and uses a probe to locate any "hot" (radioactive) lymph nodes. A "hot" node or node that looks blue is regarded as the sentinel lymph node and is removed for microscopic examination.

You need to have a lengthy discussion with your surgeon about the risk as well as the benefit associated with this procedure. The lymph node status is one of the strongest predicators for survival outcome, which is one of the benefits of undergoing the procedure. Many patients, especially young and healthy patients, want to know their risks. It offers a certain peace of mind if they know they have no lymph node involvement. Of course, as with any surgery, there are potential negative effects associated with this procedure. Potential side effects include infection, lymphedema (swelling of the limb), poor wound healing, numbness, and fluid accumulation in the surgical site, called *seroma*.

Not every melanoma patient needs this procedure. Your physician may consider many factors before recommending that you have a sentinel node biopsy. In some cases, the recommendation for sentinel node biopsy will be easily made. In other cases the decision may be difficult, and you and your physician will need to discuss the pros and cons thoroughly. Together, you will reach a plan.

Here are some basic guidelines regarding which patients do *not* need the sentinel lymph node biopsy. First, patients with stage 0 disease (melanoma in situ) do not need this procedure. For patients with stage 0 disease, the likelihood that melanoma cells have spread to the lymph nodes is very, very low. Second, patients with stage IV disease do not need lymph node biopsy. People with stage IV melanoma have metastatic disease involving the skin, lungs, or other visceral organs. The doctor can determine this by clinical exam, laboratory studies, and imaging work-ups, so biopsy of a lymph node is unnecessary. Third, many experts believe that patients with melanomas located on the trunk or extremities and whose lesions have Breslow thickness less than 1 mm (some say less than 0.75 mm) do not need sentinel lymph node biopsy. However, for patients with invasive melanoma on the head and neck region, many surgeons explore with their patients the possibility of doing sentinel lymph node biopsy.

Which Melanoma Patients Benefit Most from Sentinel Lymph Node Biopsy?

Most physicians and surgeons start discussing sentinel lymph node biopsy with their patients if the melanoma has a Breslow thickness greater than 1 mm and up to 4 mm. Most surgeons feel that sentinel lymph node biopsy is not helpful when the Breslow thickness is greater than 4 mm.

How Does Your Doctor Check for Distant Organ Involvement?

If there is lymph node involvement, the stage of disease will be changed to at least stage III. To check for possible spread of melanomas to other parts of the body, which is an indication of stage IV disease, you will be given a thorough exam.

To perform the exam, a team of specialists, including dermatologists, oncologists, surgeons, and radiologists, may be brought together. In addition to some basic checks performed by these physicians, special studies are needed for patients with thick melanomas (Breslow thickness greater than 2 mm) and for patients with known lymph node involvement.

Different specialists will focus on different areas of the body. For example, dermatologists have the most extensive training in detecting skin cancer, so the dermatologist will perform the skin exam, but a dermatologist may not listen to the lungs or feel the abdomen. An oncologist may listen to the lungs and feel the abdomen but probably will not perform the whole body skin exam.

A full skin exam is needed to check for possible metastatic disease to other skin sites. Your doctors may inspect and palpate (feel) the skin near the initial melanoma site. In addition, they may look for any nodules deep in the skin that might contain metastasis of melanoma cells. Any suspicious lesions will be biopsied. A skin metastasis looks different from a primary melanoma under the microscope. Aside from looking for skin metastases, the doctors are also looking for other primary melanomas.

In addition to the skin exam, a comprehensive physical exam may be carried out. This physical exam is very much like a routine physical exam, but the emphasis is on the lungs, liver, and skin. Your oncologists may listen to the lung area with a stethoscope. They may feel the right and left side of your abdomen, just below the ribcage, to see if there is any enlargement of the liver or spleen. They will palpate the scar at the surgical site from the excisional treatment.

In addition to performing the physical exam, your physicians will ask a series of questions to gauge your overall health. These questions will include:

- Do you feel tired? Have you lost any weight? (These questions assess your overall health status.)
- Have you recently had any persistent coughing or shortness of breath that cannot be easily explained? (These are symptoms reflecting a potential lung problem.)

- How is your overall appetite? Have you experienced nausea, vomiting, diarrhea? (These questions assess your liver and digestive system.)
- Do you have any recent history of blurry vision or intense headaches? (These questions assess your brain and eye health.)

What Blood Tests or Imaging Studies Are Needed?

There are no absolute guidelines for what types of blood work and imaging studies should be done for melanoma patients. Generally, which tests are ordered depends on the Breslow thickness of the tumor and the presence or absence of lymph node involvement. In general, for stage 0 and stage IA patients, a simple panel of blood work and an x-ray may be ordered as baseline measurements against which to compare later blood tests and x-rays, should the cancer recur or spread. However, many physicians do not order any blood tests, because this practice is not supported by evidence-based medicine. For people with stage IB to stage II melanoma, a complete blood count (CBC), basic metabolic panels, liver function test (LFT), and lactic dehydrogenase (LDH) may be ordered. For patients with a thick tumor, a CT scan of the chest, abdomen, and pelvis (groin area) may be ordered to provide a baseline record. For patients with very deep melanomas, some physicians obtain a head MRI and whole body PET scan as part of a complete work-up. Because there is no general consensus, you must discuss with the physicians who are caring for you which tests need to be done and why.

Understand Your Treatment Options

Staging is a crucial component in the decisions that are made about what treatment is appropriate for each patient. Accurate staging is therefore essential. The need for accurate staging brings us back to the importance of Step 3—having a good team of physicians caring for you. By the way, during discussions with your team, you may hear levels and stages mentioned often. Remember that Clark levels are totally different from disease stages. (I was consulted by a 31-year-old banker who had confused Clark level IV for AJCC stage IV, causing him and his family great concern. When I told him that he in fact had easily treatable stage IB disease, he was instantly relieved and now laughs about the confusion.)

Treatments are grouped into *local disease control* and *systemic treatment*. "Local control" refers to the removal of the tumor plus a rim of normal surrounding skin, if possible. The aim of this excision is to remove all of the tumor. For patients with stage III disease, which involves "positive" lymph nodes, all the lymph nodes in a specific area may be removed.

Because different treatments are needed for different stages of diseases and even for different patients with the same stage of disease (depending on their overall health and condition, for example, as well as their personal preferences), the following discussions are intended as an informational guide only. They cannot replace the consultation and medical advice offered by your own physicians. Also, modern medicine progresses at an extraordinarily fast pace. There may be cutting edge treatments available as you read this book that were not available when the book was being written and therefore are not discussed here. The bottom line? Listen to those clinical experts you trust.

The treatment options generally recommended to patients with specific stages of disease are summarized in Table 2.3. Again, the treatment options listed in this table are only a guide; the table does not replace a consultation with your doctor. Your physician's advice may not match the summary recommendations because he or she knows your specific condition well and can design a better treatment plan for you. *The discussion that follows does not replace the advice and treatment plans offered by your doctors.*

Stage 0

Patients in this stage have melanoma in situ; the melanoma cells have not penetrated beyond the epidermis. The treatment action is relatively straightforward: remove the tumor and a standard surgical margin of 5 mm. "Standard surgical margin" refers to the amount of normal surrounding skin tissue that needs to be removed.

Table 2.3. Melanoma Treatment Recommendations

Stage	Surgical Treatment	Systemic Treatment
Stage 0	Excision with a 5 mm margin	No
Stage IA	Excision with a 1 cm margin	No
Stage IB to II	Excision with a 1 to 2 cm margin depending on the Breslow thickness	Consider sentinel lymph node biopsy
Stage III	Excision and lymph node dissection	Consider: adjuvant alpha interferon, vaccine trial, clinical trial of chemotherapy, radiation, isolated limb perfusion
Stage IV	Consider resection of individual or limited lesions	Consider: adjuvant interferon, vaccine trial, clinical trial of chemotherapy, radiation, isolated limb perfusion/infusion

Stage I

The treatment for stage I melanoma consists of a standard excision of the tumor along with a standard surgical margin of 1 cm. Depending on the Breslow thickness, ulceration status, and location of the melanoma, your surgeon may discuss with you the need for sentinel lymph node biopsy, which would be done at the same time as the excision of the tumor. Currently, there is no consensus of opinion on which patients should have sentinel lymph node biopsy. In general, there seems to be an agreement that sentinel lymph node biopsy should be performed for patients with melanomas larger than 1 mm in Breslow thickness. However, some surgeons urge that sentinel lymph node biopsy be performed for patients with melanomas of 0.75 mm or deeper. *You need to talk about this with your physician.*

Here is the description by one melanoma patient, Gloria, of her experience with the standard excision procedure.

My melanoma was found by my dermatologist during an annual skin exam. Right then he biopsied the worrisome lesion, which was on my right arm, and one week later he telephoned me with the diagnosis of melanoma. I was very worried. He explained the biopsy results and said that the lesion needed to be removed, and soon. I was glad when he told me that the melanoma was relatively thin. It had a Breslow thickness of 0.25 mm. I did not really understand what that meant at the time. Another thing I remember is my dermatologist urging me not to go online and do too much research. He warned me that some of the information on the Web might scare me.

On the day of surgery, I was rather nervous. I arrived in his office 30 minutes prior to my scheduled appointment. His secretary asked me to fill out a questionnaire. Soon, a nurse brought me into a procedure room. The room was about 10 by 12 feet, clean and organized. It was not like those operating rooms you see on television or what I had imagined. Next, the nurse asked me a series of questions regarding my health, past medical history, allergies, and current medications. She took my blood pressure and measured my heart rate. She was kind and gentle. Before leaving the room, the nurse gave me a gown to change into.

It was not long before my dermatologist walked into the room. He was wearing a blue hospital "scrub" outfit instead of the usual white coat. He shook my hand and asked how I was feeling. Then he explained the diagnosis again and described the procedure he would be doing. He said that the surgery was fairly straightforward but that there were potential risks, including pain, infection, bleeding, scarring, swelling, and numbness, and that there was the possibility of recurrence of the melanoma. His explanation was clear, but it also made me feel more anxious. When he asked if I had any questions, I shook my head and signed a consent form that allowed him to do the surgery.

I lay back in a very comfortable exam chair. The nurse positioned the chair in a fully reclined position and offered me a pillow for my head. Next the doctor marked the site on my right arm and cleaned the area with alcohol. The smell and cold sensation made me a little anxious. He told me that he would give me a shot to numb the area. I only felt a tiny sting when he gave me the shot. I did not feel any pain after that. My doctor was constantly talking to me and letting me know what he was doing, and that helped me not to worry as much. Soon, my arm felt like it was getting swollen. The doctor assured me that that was a normal sensation.

Next I heard him opening his tray of surgical instruments, but I did not see them. A few sterile towels were placed on my right arm, and he cleaned the area again, with some different fluid this time. The nurse asked me what music I would like to hear. I thought to myself that I didn't care; anything would be fine. Seeing my hesitation, she suggested something soothing and I agreed. I felt my doctor and his assistant touching my arm as the nurse started the music. Next, the doctor looked at me and said, "Gloria, we are doing well. I already removed the tumor."

Naturally I was surprised that it was gone already. Next I felt some tugging sensations in my right arm and slowly felt that the arm was getting tighter, less like it was swollen. However, I did not feel any pain. My doctor reassured me that everything was going well, and 5 to 10 minutes later, he told me that the whole procedure was over. I was relieved.

My doctor gave me some instruction on how to care for the wound, the place where he'd removed the lesion, and he shook my hand before leaving the room. His nurse then cleaned the area around the wound and put a bandage over the area. She then went over the wound care instructions again and gave me a written instruction sheet. She said that I could take some Tylenol if I had pain, but no Advil or ibuprofen, because both of those medicines can increase the risk of bleeding. I got off the comfortable chair, changed back into my clothes, and thanked everyone in the office.

Overall, my experience was great. There was some minor pain that night. I took two Tylenol and applied some ice over the area. It didn't hurt after that. Two weeks later, I went back to the dermatologist's office. He took out the suture and told me that all the tumor had been removed. I felt like a heavy weight had been lifted off my shoulders.

Stage IIA with Breslow Thickness of <2 mm

Standard excision of the melanoma along with a margin of 1 cm is commonly recommended for patients with stage IIA melanoma with tumors less than 2 millimeters thick. In general, sentinel lymph node biopsy is also performed, at the time of the tumor excision.

Stage IIA with Breslow Thickness >2 mm, Stage IIB, and IIC

Usual treatment for these diagnoses is standard excision of the melanoma tumor with a surgical margin of 2 cm of normal tissue. Sentinel lymph node biopsy may also be performed at the time of the excision. However, many clinicians feel that the value of sentinel lymph node biopsy for melanomas with Breslow thickness greater than 4 mm is very limited. Your physicians may discuss adding treatment involving interferon (discussed below under "Immuno-therapy") as an adjuvant therapy, an additional treatment given af-ter the initial cancer has been treated, to help prevent the cancer from coming back.

Stage III and Stage IV

Systemic therapy may be needed in addition to excision for pa-tients with stage III and stage IV disease. Systemic therapy is treatment that travels through the bloodstream to reach all parts of the body. Your physician may also recommend adjuvant therapy, to help prevent a recurrence.

Generally your medical oncologist (rather than a surgical or ra-diation oncologist) will discuss with you the risks and benefits of any systemic treatments suggested for you. A face-to-face consulta-tion is necessary for you to understand the treatment plans and so you can ask questions. You may be given a great deal of informa-tion. It is a good idea to bring someone with you for your oncology consultation. A family member or friend can listen along with you and take notes, and you should review the discussion with that per-son later. The notes from the consultation will help you think about what you want to do before committing to any treatment options. Getting second or third opinions with other specialists in different medical centers is a good idea, but these consultations must happen without delay. During your discussions with these physicians, keep in mind that statistics from research studies do not necessarily predict how a treatment will work in any specific individual.

The following section will briefly discuss some of the systemic treatments for melanoma. Some of these medications are approved by the U.S. Food and Drug Administration (FDA) for use in the treatment of melanoma, but many of the drugs are used to treat advanced melanoma even though they have not been approved by the FDA for this purpose; they have been approved for other purposes. This practice of using FDA-approved drugs but for purposes for which they are not approved by the FDA is called *off-label drug use,* and it is a common practice in medicine. Physicians make these treatment decisions based on their clinical experience and data gathered by researchers who are studying particular drugs in treating other diseases. In addition, there are also many ongoing clinical trials testing unusual drugs or combinations of drugs.

Unfortunately, most of the systemic treatments have produced excellent results in only a small percentage of melanoma patients.

Immunotherapy

Immunotherapy is a category of treatments that aim to boost the body's immune system to help it find, target, and destroy the melanoma cells.

Interferon-alfa. This drug is approved by the FDA as an adjuvant treatment for patients with stage IIB and stage III melanoma. Clinical trials have shown that this drug, which is a manufactured substance that is similar in chemical structure to a protein naturally produced in the body (interferon-alpha), may improve the five-year survival chances for patients with stage III disease. However, it is important to point out that many patients experience multiple side effects, and that the drug is not as effective as we had hoped. (See next paragraph for more about interferon.)

Tumor necrosis factor. This substance is naturally produced in the body. Both tumor necrosis factor and the natural protein interferon-alpha are produced by the lymphocytes, a subclass of white blood cells. The production of interferon and tumor necrosis factor initiates a cascade of activities in which the body's innate immune cells are activated to search and destroy tumor cells. The drug interferon-alfa is approved by the FDA for treating melanoma, but tumor necrosis factor is not.

Melanoma vaccines. Vaccines for melanoma work through the same immune mechanism just described above. They are thought to be a promising treatment for patients with stage III and stage IV disease. Unlike the flu vaccines used to keep people from contracting influenza, melanoma vaccines stimulate the body's immune system to kill disease after it has appeared, improving the immune cells' ability to search and destroy tumor cells. A number of melanoma vaccines are being tested in academic medical centers. As of 2011, no vaccine had attained FDA approval.

Interleukin-2. This is another naturally produced substance that can boost the innate immune cells' ability to destroy melanoma cells. This drug is approved by the FDA for this use.

Chemotherapy

In chemotherapy, generally a number of drugs are given together in combination. Various "cocktails" of drugs have been used to treat patients with stage IV disease.

Decarbazine (DTIC). This drug is delivered intravenously. It was approved by the FDA for patients with stage IV melanoma in the 1970s.

Temozolomide. Although this drug works through a similar mechanism as DTIC, many oncologists prefer temozolomide because it has fewer negative side effects and can be given by mouth instead of into a vein. Also, because this drug can penetrate into the brain, it can target any metastatic tumors in the brain. Although this drug is often prescribed to treat other stage III and stage IV cancers, it is not FDA approved for melanoma treatment.

In general, neither of these drugs is optimal for patients with lung or other visceral organ involvement.

Isolated Limb Perfusion

Some patients with advanced stages of melanoma on the lower limbs with skin metastases may be offered the option to receive isolated limb perfusion treatment. This procedure aims to deliver a high dose of chemotherapy to the tumors in the legs or arms while preventing the drugs from reaching the other parts of the body. During the procedure, the surgeon places a tourniquet on the affected limb where the melanoma tumor is located. The tourniquet prevents the drugs from leaking into other parts of the body. A catheter is placed in a vein in the same limb. Blood is drawn away from the limb and then passed through an apparatus that slowly adds oxygen and chemotherapy drugs to the blood. The blood, carrying this high dose of chemotherapy drugs, is then returned to the affected limb. The procedure takes more than an hour to complete. Complications include pain, swelling, nerve damage, and ulceration of the skin. In selected types of patients, this treatment can reduce the size of or completely eradicate tumors.

Radiation

In general, radiation is not used as a curative treatment for melanoma. This treatment modality is usually adopted as an adjuvant treatment, to prevent recurrence of the disease after primary treatment. Radiation oncologists are the specialists who plan and deliver this treatment. A complete course of radiation treatment is often divided into sessions spanning weeks or months. The common side effects include inflammation of the irradiated area. The inflammation can resemble a severe sunburn, and the irradiated skin can break down, resulting in painful erosion or ulceration. Moisturizers and antibiotic lotions may be used to soothe and heal the area.

Step 5. Understand Survival Rate and Prognosis

Prognosis means the probable outcome of a disease. This prediction can be measured in terms of cure rate, remission rate, recurrence rate, or survival rate. Although all of these measurements are valuable to researchers and to clinicians for monitoring the progress of treatments, I will focus on only the overall survival rate. Survival rate depends on the AJCC stage of the disease, patients' response to the treatments, patients' general health, and other factors.

Before I discuss the survival rates for different stages of melanoma, I want to highlight the following points. First, the survival data presented below come from research studies. These are the same survival data quoted in many medical textbooks. The data were compiled from studies of large populations of patients with known stages of melanoma and who had had long-term follow-up. These data represent the best *estimate*, based on the historical data, of patient survival rates.

There are many factors to keep in mind when looking at these survival data. First, these are predictions of the survival outcomes of groups of patients with similar stages of disease. This does *not* mean that all patients in a particular group will have the same outcome. The data presented are the average survival rates for groups of similar patients. *There will always be exceptions in any statistical model.* I have taken care of patients with very advanced stages of disease who have defied the statistical prediction and are still doing very well decades after their initial diagnosis and treatment.

Second, the survival data were generated by melanoma studies done several years ago, when our understanding and treatment of the disease was not as advanced as it is today. Modern science and clinical research are advancing at a breathtaking pace. New treatment regimens have been, and are continually being, developed to combat this cancer. Although the survival rate for advanced stages of melanoma can be disheartening, it is entirely possible for modern medicine to alter the course of even late-stage disease.

Third, the validity of any prediction model depends on the size of the patient samples. A good question to ask about any research study is, How many patients were in the study? If the prediction is based on a small number of patients, it may be less accurate than a model generated from a large sample of patients. The survival data presented below are based on 38,918 patients, a large sample; but for stage III and stage IV disease, the survival data are based on only 3,307 and 7,972 patients, respectively.

Table 2.4. Survival Data Based on the 2002 AJCC Staging System

Stage	Number of Patients	Survival Percentages	
		5 Years	10 Years
O	*	100	100
IA	4,510	95	88
IB	1,380	91	83
	3,285	89	79
IIA	958	77	64
	1,717	79	64
IIB	1,523	63	51
	563	67	54
IIC	978	45	32
IIIA	382	63–70	57–63
IIIB	543	46–59	36–48
IIIC	603	24–29	15–24
IV	(Skin involvement)		
	179	19	16
	(Lung involvement)		
	186	7	3
	(All other organs)		
	793	10	6
Total	**17,600**		

*Data not employed in AJCC system.

The survival rates of patients with different stages of melanoma are summarized in Table 2.4. Only five-year and ten-year survival data are presented in this table. The numbers under those two columns indicate the percentage of patients in each disease stage subgroup of studied participants who were still living at the end of five or ten years after diagnosis of melanoma. For example, the survival rates for patients with stage IA disease at five years and ten years are 95 percent and 88 percent, respectively. In contrast, for patients with stage IVB disease (metastatic melanoma to the lung), the survival rates at five and ten years are 7 percent and 3 percent, respectively.

The table illustrates, first, that not all melanomas are equal. For stage 0 (in situ melanoma) disease, the five-year and ten-year survival rates are nearly 100 percent (so near that it can be reported as 100% in the table). For thin melanomas, with Breslow thickness less than 1 mm, the survival rate is also excellent. Patients with early stages of melanoma should be relieved to know that people with early melanoma have an excellent survival rate.

Second, the table shows that melanoma is a very dangerous type of skin cancer. The aggressive nature of melanoma is demonstrated by the low survival rate in patients with advanced stages of the disease. Aggressive and timely intervention by a team of clinical experts is crucial in the fight to cure a patient.

Before closing this chapter on the five steps for surviving the "mad rush" phase of melanoma, I want to share the following thoughts, which I hope will provide comfort and support to those in an advanced stage of the disease. The survival data for stage III and IV patients can be disheartening, but it is very important to remember that statistics can be misleading. You are a unique individual; you are not a random number. The statistical data are created to help physicians choose the optimal treatment options for patients and estimate survival outcomes. The key word is "estimate." There are countless examples of cancer patients who defied statistics, fought their diseases, and experienced remission or have been cured. I have cared for patients who survived advanced stages of melanoma, and I have heard stories from colleagues about patients who beat the odds in the face of dire statistics. In all of these cases, patients found reasons to hope, to fight, and to live.

These success stories also teach us that treatments that failed or were inadequate in a majority of cases actually can help certain patients. More importantly, modern medicine does not stand still. We in the scientific and medical communities are working constantly to unlock new treatments for melanoma. We learn from our failures and we learn from our successes. While writing this book I learned about some very exciting new treatment paradigms that could alter the survival statistics. I sincerely believe that these new treatment modalities will prove to be effective as they undergo additional clinical trials.

Lastly, what the patient brings to the therapeutic process makes a difference. Physicians provide guidance and treatment, and patients need to enlist family, friends, and other health care givers to provide support. Keeping your spirit positive and determined and keeping your mind strong can help you beat the disease.

3. The "Marathon" Phase

Surviving Melanoma

The "mad rush" phase of dealing with melanoma is a high-pressure, fast-paced time when most patients feel as if they are shuttling from doctor to doctor for work-ups and treatment. Many patients feel a sense of chaos and loss of control. The five-step guide in Chapter 2 aims to provide the necessary vocabulary and background information to help people navigate their way through this intense phase.

As I mentioned in the Preface, after successful treatment and passing through the "mad rush" phase, many patients initially feel a sense of relief. Soon, however, they develop new questions and concerns. As they learn more about the disease, they want to know: Do I need any additional treatment? How can I protect myself from developing additional melanomas in the future? Will my children or other family members develop melanoma? These questions can linger for months or years. In fact, this is a natural part of the process, because patients have been actively engaged in learning new information, and they become accustomed to asking questions and uncovering facts. Moreover, a diagnosis of melanoma often can change an individual's attitude, behavior, and lifestyle. Thus, I have dubbed the second part of the the melanoma experience the "marathon," reflecting the ongoing journey.

The discussion in this chapter is divided into the following sections:

- "Medical Follow-Up," about ongoing medical care
- "Who Is at Risk for Developing Melanoma?" about whether you and family members may be at risk

- "Preventing Melanoma," a discussion of lifestyle and behavior changes to prevent additional melanomas from developing and to catch any new ones at an early stage
- "Medical Developments," which describes some of the new technologies

Medical Follow-Up

Why Do You Need Continual Follow-Up Examinations?

The benefit of medical follow-up immediately after surgery or other treatment is obvious. Your physicians want to make sure that the excision wound is healing and that you have tolerated the treatment well. But continuing follow-ups are also needed, even long after the surgery or treatment has been completed. There are many reasons for these later follow-up visits. First, you need to make sure that the original melanoma has not recurred or come back. For patients who had intermediate or advanced stages of melanoma, the continuing follow-up is needed to make certain that there are no melanomas in other parts of the body. History, physical exam, and laboratory and imaging studies may be ordered to stay on top of the situation.

Second, follow-ups provide a good opportunity to detect any new melanomas at an early stage. People with a personal history of melanoma are at a higher risk for developing new melanoma, especially in the first five years after the first incidence. Some studies estimate the risk that a person with a prior personal history of melanoma will develop a new melanoma at nine times higher than the risk of melanoma in the general public.

Which Specialist or Specialists Should
You See for Follow-Ups?

Depending on the stage of your melanoma, you may need various specialists for your ongoing care. Dermatologists focus on the detection of new skin cancers. Follow-up with a dermatologist for a total skin exam, to check for additional skin cancers, is recommended at least once a year. Some patients need quarterly follow-ups with a total skin exam during the first few years after treatment.

For patients who had early stage melanoma, the role of medical oncologists and surgeons may be limited, and some melanoma patients may never need the care of these specialists. For patients who had an advanced stage of the disease, medical oncologists and surgeons will play a more active role in the follow-up process. Surgeons will focus on the scars and other surgery-related issues. Medical oncologists and internists tend to focus on overall health status. You should follow up with your primary care or family doctor to monitor your other health issues.

How Frequently Should You Have Follow-Up Exams?

There are no specific guidelines issued by medical committees on the optimal frequency of follow-up exams. The frequency largely depends on the stage of the disease and number of years that have passed since the original diagnosis of melanoma. Patients who had advanced stages of the disease need to have much more frequent follow-up checks. Patients whose diagnosis and treatment were recent also need to have frequent follow-ups. As a general rule, any person who has had a melanoma should be seen by a physician at least once a year.

What Should You Expect during Follow-Up Visits?

Your physicians will ask about your overall health, current medications, and the status of any other medical conditions. Specifically, they may ask about any weight loss or weight gain and symptoms associated with specific organs. These pieces of information are known as (1) history of present illness and (2) past medical history. Asking these questions helps the physicians detect any signs that the melanoma has appeared in other parts of the body. For example, patients with persistent cough may prompt a suspicion that the melanoma has spread to the lungs.

In addition to taking a history and asking questions, the physicians will perform physical exams. The scope of the exams will vary depending on the specialist you are seeing. For example, dermatologists will focus on the skin, performing a total body skin exam, including the scalp and the bottoms of your feet. In addition, they will focus on the melanoma scars, checking for recurrence at the original site. Medical oncologists and general internists will listen to your lungs, heart, and abdomen with a stethoscope, and will palpate your abdomen to check for any potential enlargement of your liver or spleen.

Who Is at Risk for Developing Melanoma?

Most melanoma survivors want to know the answers to this question. Most of my patients are concerned about whether they are at risk for developing additional melanomas and whether their immediate relatives, especially their children, may develop melanomas. The answer to these questions lies in understanding the specific risk factors associated with developing melanoma. In fact, we now know that individuals with certain genetic backgrounds, patterns of environmental exposure, and family histories are at higher risk. For those individuals, extra caution is needed to try to prevent melanomas.

What Is Your Skin Color?

Hair color, eye color, and skin color are determined by genetics—by the genes we inherit from our parents. Individuals with a certain characteristic appearance (called a phenotype) are more susceptible to developing melanomas. In general, people with blond or red hair, a fair complexion, and/or numerous freckles have a high lifetime risk of developing melanoma. Those individuals tend to burn easily and do not tan. To categorize individual differences, dermatologists have defined six skin types (called Fitzpatrick Skin Type), ranging from light to dark (see Table 3.1). Although people with any skin type can develop melanomas, individuals with skin types I, II, and III are at higher risk than people with the other skin types.

Table 3.1. Fitzpatrick Skin Types

Skin Type	Sunburning	Tanning	Other Characteristics
I	Always burns	Never tans	Pale white skin, red or blond hair, blue or hazel eyes
II	Burns easily	Tans poorly	Fair skin
III	Burns	Tans after initial burn	Darker white skin
IV	Burns minimally	Tans easily	Light brown skin
V	Rarely burns	Tans darkly and easily	Brown skin
VI	Never burns	Tans quickly	Dark brown or dark skin

How Much Sun Exposure Have You Had?

Individuals with a history of intense and intermittent UV (ultraviolet light) exposure are at a high lifetime risk of developing melanoma. The UV exposure can come from the sun or from artificial sources such as tanning booths. UV radiation can be divided into short UV waves (UVB) and long UV waves (UVA). Both types of ultraviolet radiation can produce cellular and tissue damage. UVB causes direct damage to the DNA in the cells, and UVA interacts with organelles (structures) in the tissue and generates oxygen radicals which indirectly damage the DNA. Individuals with a history of blistering sunburns, especially at an early age, have significantly higher risks for developing melanoma.

What Is Your Personal and Family History?

Individuals with prior personal history or family history of melanoma are at higher risk for developing melanoma. In addition, individuals with many atypical (dysplastic) moles (nevi) have a higher risk. Table 3.2 presents the estimated increase in risk for various melanoma risk factors. Some of the statistics are shocking.

Table 3.2. Risk Factors for Developing Melanomas

Risk Factors	Estimated Relative Risk*
Atypical nevi, prior melanoma and familial melanoma	500
Large number of atypical nevi, familial melanoma and no prior melanoma	148
Atypical nevi, no prior melanoma or familial melanoma	7–27
Many nevi (more than 50)	7–54
Giant congenital melanocytic nevi	101
Personal history of melanoma	9
History of melanoma in first-degree blood relatives	8
Immunosuppression	2–8
Red or blond hair and blue eyes	1–6

Estimated relative risk means the number of times more likely a person with these characteristics is to develop melanoma than the average person is.

For example, compared to the risk in the general public, the risk of developing melanomas for individuals with many moles (more than 50) is 7 to 54 times higher. Individuals with some atypical moles but no personal or family history of melanomas are 7 to 27 times more likely to develop melanoma than people in the general population.

The most stunning statistic is the increase in risk for persons with atypical moles, prior personal history of melanoma, *and* a family history of melanoma. These individuals' likelihood of developing another melanoma is 500 times higher than that of the general public. That is why individuals with many moles, atypical moles, prior personal history of melanoma, or family history of melanoma should have close follow-up. A full-body skin exam at least once a year is needed. Also, because family history of melanoma is a risk factor, if you have melanoma, please tell your immediate relatives (children, siblings, and parents) that they should have at least a baseline skin examination. By telling them, you may save the life of someone you love.

Do You Have Large Moles that Were Present at Birth?

Individuals with "giant" congenital moles have a higher risk of developing melanoma than does the general public (*congenital* means "at birth"). "Giant" congenital moles are defined as moles that are larger than 20 cm in diameter in an adult (they grow as the body grows). Although melanomas can develop in small or medium-sized congenital moles, the occurrence of melanomas in them is much lower. Persons who were born with a large congenital mole generally should be monitored closely by their health care providers for signs of melanoma.

Preventing Melanoma

There are two categories of melanoma prevention: primary prevention and secondary prevention. *Primary prevention* focuses on keeping the melanoma from occurring in the first place. It involves our perception and behavior with regard to excessive UV exposure. You can't control your family history, your skin type, or moles present at birth, but you can exert considerable control over your UV exposure. Many scientific studies have demonstrated that intermittent and intense sun exposure plays a major role in the development of melanoma. Hence, anything you can do to reduce harmful UV exposure from the sun or any other UV source may help prevent skin cancers.

Secondary prevention focuses on early detection of the disease. As I have stressed in this book, only early diagnosis followed by prompt removal of the melanomas can ensure a good outcome. Physicians, especially dermatologists, play an important role, but many clinical studies have shown that most melanomas are first spotted by the patients or their family members or friends. Hence, *you* can detect melanomas on yourself and on your friends and family members.

Now we'll explore some of the strategies you can use in both primary and secondary prevention.

Primary Prevention: Avoid Excessive UV Exposure

The main goal is to reduce the total amount of ultraviolet ray exposure, whether it comes from the sun or from any other source, such as a tanning booth. Here are four layers of protection you should employ, in order of importance:

1. Avoid excessive sun exposure and stay away from tanning booths.
2. Seek shade.
3. Wear protective clothing and hats.
4. Use sunscreens.

Sun avoidance. Staying out of the sun is the best way to reduce UV exposure. However, total avoidance is not possible and may be also detrimental to our health. In fact, there are a number of health benefits associated with sun exposure. Outdoor activities promote an active and healthy lifestyle, for example. Sunshine brightens our mood. (Many patients tell me, "Dr. Wang, I love the sun. It makes me feel good.") Recent scientific studies have suggested that vitamin D, produced in the skin after sun exposure, reduces the risk of colon and breast cancers. Although the best sources of vitamin D are food and vitamin supplements, we still need to obtain a certain level of UV exposure from the sun to make enough vitamin D.

So, complete sun avoidance is not possible and not recommended. You should not feel guilty the next time you are out in the sun; with some precautions you can enjoy your outdoor fun with your family and friends. One kind of UV exposure you can and should completely avoid. You should *never use a tanning booth* (more on the danger of tanning booths below). Strive to cut back on the total amount of UV exposure you get. Avoid the peak UV radiation hours of 10 a.m. to 4 p.m. The UV rays are most intense during this period.

Seek shade. Whenever you are sitting or lying outdoors for an extended period, use shade structures, such as awnings, trees, and umbrellas. Staying in the shade allows you to enjoy being outdoors while still getting the protection you need from UV radiation. When you are barbecuing or lying on the beach, seek available shade and provide shade for yourself (as with a beach umbrella).

Hats and clothing. In addition to avoiding the most intense rays of the sun and seeking shade, you need to cover yourself with a hat and protective clothing. I advise my patients to wear UV protective clothing and hats. I prefer hats and clothing over sunscreens. Unlike sunscreens, clothing is not greasy and you don't need to reapply it. Shaded structures may be difficult to find in some situations, but hats and clothing can protect you anywhere, as long as you remember to wear them.

Some of my patients complain that long sleeve pants and shirts are too hot to wear in the summer. Good point!—and I have an answer: there is an increasing number of specialty clothing manufacturers (for example, Coolibar and Sun Precautions' Solumbra line) that produce lightweight, cool, breezy, and fashionable clothing designed to block UV rays from the sun. This clothing is made from special fabric with close weave. These clothing lines satisfy everyone, including the fashion conscious. You need to wear a wide brim hat that shades your ears, cheeks, nose, and a part of your neck. A baseball cap doesn't provide adequate shade, and UV rays penetrate the holes in a straw hat. If you wear one of these hats, you are not getting adequate coverage. Please visit www.melanomapictures.org and the "Melanoma Prevention" section for samples of effective protective clothing.

Sunscreens. I put sunscreen fourth (and last) on the list of primary prevention strategies for two reasons. First, sunscreen is less helpful in photoprotection (protection from UV rays) than seeking shade or wearing protective clothing and hats. Second, sunscreen is what most people think of *first* when they think about sun protection. At the end of most consultations with my patients, I talk to them about the importance of protecting themselves against UV exposure. Almost inevitably, the first question I get back from the patient is, "Which sunscreens should I use?" Before I give my recommendations, I would like to highlight some of the problems with sunscreens. Understanding these problems will help you see why I think sunscreens are inferior to other protection strategies.

First, *most people do not use enough sunscreen to achieve the desired protection.* SPF is the well-known measure used to rate the efficacy of any sunscreen. It stands for "sun protection factor," although this definition may be soon changed to "sunburn protection factor" (as I discuss below). All sunscreen products have an SPF number, such as SPF 30 or SPF 55. Unfortunately, for most users, the actual degree of SPF protection received is much less than that stated on the product label. For example, a sunscreen product with an SPF of 30 may only provide an SPF 10 in the real-life setting. How can this be?

The SPF value of each sunscreen product is measured in a laboratory using human subjects for each test. In the test, a concentration of 2 milligrams of sunscreen for each square centimeter of skin is applied to each person's back, and then the testing is done and an SPF score is assigned to the product. But for the average adult to achieve that concentration of sunscreen, he or she needs to use 1.4 ounces (1 shot glassful) of sunscreen to cover the whole body at each application! Since most sunscreens on the market are packaged in 6 to 8 ounce tubes, this means that an average-sized adult will use up a tube of sunscreen in only 3 to 5 applications.

Most people use much less than the desired amount. For most families, a tube of sunscreen is used many times in a summer season. Sometimes, it will even last until the next summer. Studies have shown that most people use a concentration of only 0.5 to 1 mg/cm^2 of sunscreen at each application (and some use less). That's one-quarter to one-half the amount they should be using. Hence, in real-life settings, the degree of SPF protection is dramatically lower than predicted on sunscreen packaging. That's how a sunscreen product with an SPF of 30 comes to provide protection equivalent to an SPF of as little as 10 in the real-life setting.

Second, *the SPF label is misleading.* As mentioned above, currently the SPF designation stands for sun protection factor. Judging by the name, you would assume that the label gives an indication of the protection from the entire UV spectrum. In fact, SPF is designed to measure predominately the UVB (290 to 320 nm wave length) portion of the UV spectrum. UVB is the main culprit for producing sunburn. The SPF measurement does not give any indication about the degree of protection from UVA radiation (320 to 400 nm wave length). Scientific studies have shown that both UVA and UVB play important roles in causing skin cancers. UVB produces direct DNA damage, causing the nucleotides in your DNA to crosslink to each other. In contrast, UVA can induce indirect damage to the tissue. Currently, the FDA is proposing standards for measuring UVA as well.

Third, *most sunscreens on the market do not provide adequate UVA protection*. Although many brands claim that their products offer a broad spectrum of both UVB and UVA protection, the degree of UVA protection varies significantly from one product to another. As of 2009, no regulations exist regarding standards for UVA protection. A test I conducted on the thirteen best-selling sunscreens in the United States was published in the *Journal of the American Academy of Dermatology* in December 2008. Of the thirteen products I tested, only five met the high-protection standard in the FDA's proposed guideline ("proposed guideline" because there were no official testing standards at the time of our laboratory study). The other eight products offered only medium protection from UVA rays.

What is the problem with inadequate UVA protection? The most obvious problem is that you may use a sunscreen with a very high SPF label (such as 85) and believe that you are well protected from the whole range of UV rays. In fact, you may be receiving only good (not excellent) protection from the UVB radiation and no or little protection from the UVA rays. A sunscreen with high SPF may prevent you from being burned, and it may cause you actually to stay out in the sun longer. The end result is that you may inadvertently be receiving a disproportionally large amount of UVA rays.

Sunscreens are one part of a sun protection routine, but I want everyone to understand the shortcomings of sunscreens and to follow the instructions for proper use given in Table 3.3. Below is a list of sunscreens I can recommend as of spring 2010. Please visit www.melanomapictures.org for updates to this list. All of these

Table 3.3 Sunscreen Instructions

---

1. Apply sunscreen before you go outdoors, ideally 20 minutes before going outdoors. But if you forget to put on sunscreen before going outdoors, you need to apply sunscreen when you are outside. This might seem to go without saying, but several of my patients have told me that they decided not to apply any sunscreen after they were already outside and realized that they had forgotten to put on sunscreen before leaving the house. You need to take the sunscreen with you anyway, so you can reapply it periodically.

Applying sunscreen is important for everyone in the family, including mothers. Far too often, mothers are the ones who remind their husbands to use sunscreen and who put sunscreen on the children. If you put sunscreen on everyone else *after* you are already outdoors, by the time you apply sunscreen to yourself, you may already have been exposed to the sun without any UV protection for 20 to 30 minutes.

2. Use a generous amount. For an average-sized adult, the appropriate amount is approximately 1.4 ounces, or a shot glassful amount.

3. Remember to reapply the sunscreen again, generously. If you are sweating profusely or are in contact with water, you need to reapply sunscreen at least every two hours.

4. Remember to use sunscreens every day, even on overcast days. You can use a moisturizer with broad spectrum UV coverage (both UVB and UVA coverage). This simple action of using a moisturizer can prevent skin cancers and slow down signs of aging. UV exposure is the main agent for causing uneven pigmentations or blotches on the face, and it can degrade the collagens, making the skin wrinkle and sag.

---

products are recommended based on the most recent scientific studies.

> Banana Boat Sunwear daily sunblock lotion
> Coppertone Ultraguard sunscreen lotion (SPF 50)
> Coppertone Water Babies sunscreen lotion (SPF 50)
> Neutrogena Ultra Sheer Dry-Touch Sunblock with Helioplex (SPF 55)
> La Roche Posay Anthelios SX
> La Roche Posay Anthelios Cream with Mexoryl SX and Mexoryl XL (SPF 40)
> Coppertone Continuous Sports Spray (SPF 30)

Secondary Prevention: Detecting Melanoma at an Early Stage

Primary prevention involves preventing and reducing exposure to UV radiation. Secondary prevention, on the other hand, focuses on the early detection of melanomas. Early detection is the key to a good survival outcome. Here are the three keys to detection:

> Get periodic examinations from a physician.
> Perform regular self-examinations.
> Pay attention to symptoms.

Have Regular Total-Body Skin Examinations
Follow a regular schedule of total-body skin examinations with your physicians, preferably including a dermatologist. Dermatologists are by far the best-trained and most-skilled physicians at diagnosing melanomas and nonmelanoma skin cancers. Even among dermatologists there are some who have more expertise than others in diagnosing and treating skin cancers, especially melanomas. Dermatologists without expertise may overtreat or undertreat moles that are potentially cancerous, and neither overtreatment nor undertreatment is ideal. To help you find a dermatologist most skilled in handling melanoma, I will describe some of my and other melanoma specialists' approaches to caring for high-risk melanoma patients. You might consider looking for a specialist who follows all or most of these practices.

The total-body skin exam is the first line of defense. The reason for this is simple. Melanoma can occur almost *anywhere* on the skin, and in order to detect it, we need to look for it. I take every possible measure to ensure the comfort, privacy, and modesty of our patients. The patient is asked to remove all clothing except for underwear, and for women, bra. A robe is provided. If the patient is chilly, our staff may offer a warm blanket or set the thermostat higher to warm the room. I always follow the same routine for each exam. I start the exam at the right hand and right arm, then switch to the left hand and left arm. Then I focus on the back, chest, and abdomen, in that sequence. After the upper body, I turn my attention to the thighs, lower legs, feet, toes, and toenails. Lastly, I examine the face and the scalp. The systematic and consistent ap-

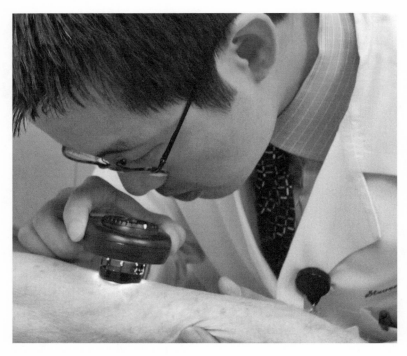

Figure 3.1. A dermoscope being used during a skin examination.

proach is important, to avoid skipping any parts of the body. The mouth, genitals, and female breasts are not examined unless the patient specifically requests an examination in these areas.

I use a dermoscope. A dermoscope is a hand-held microscope-like device (see Figure 3.1) that illuminates and magnifies structures that are not visible to the naked eye. Although the device is rather simple, interpreting what one sees with a dermoscope requires experience and knowledge. In the hands of experts, dermoscopy can significantly increase the diagnostic accuracy and diagnostic confidence of melanoma—by more than 20 percent. Many lesions look very worrisome in a naked eye exam but appear completely normal under dermoscopic examination. Using the dermoscope, I can reassure my patients in a few seconds' time, and tell them that the questionable lesion is fine and no biopsy is needed. Of course, there are times when dermoscopy confirms my initial concerns. (When the concern is confirmed, I perform a biopsy immediately.)

I use total-body cutaneous photographs when following some of my high-risk melanoma patients. Many of my patients have more than 100 moles, and some of these moles look like melanomas. They are asymmetric in shape, have irregular borders, are larger than 6 mm, and have multiple colors. Some have a history of significant changes. In other words, they display the ABCDEs of melanoma (more about this below) and are causes for concern. Some of these patients also have a personal and family history of melanoma, both of which are risk factors for developing melanoma. In keeping track of all these worrisome moles, total-body photography is very helpful.

In this approach, a set of baseline digital photographs of the entire body is taken by a professional medical photographer. The photos are captured in very high resolution. The digital photographs are stored in a secure computer server. At each visit, as I perform the skin exam, I compare the moles with the digital photos. The total-body photographs make it possible for us to track changes in the moles. Using this system, we can detect minute changes and spot new moles. The total-body photographs also can serve as a useful tool for patients when they perform their self-exams. Some of my patients receive a large book of color prints and a CD containing the clinical images of their total-body photographs. They can use this book at home during their self-exams, to compare the baseline pictures with the current appearance of their moles.

I sometimes use sequential short-term digital clinical and dermoscopic photos (taken with a camera attached to a dermoscope) for detailed monitoring of worrisome moles. Sometimes it is very difficult to tell whether lesions are benign or malignant, but biopsy may not be appropriate, for various reasons. In these cases, rather than performing a biopsy, I may choose to take close-up clinical and dermoscopic photos of the lesions; then I have the patient return in three to six months and I reexamine the lesions and take another set of close-up clinical and dermoscopic photos of the same lesions. The images are then displayed on a high-resolution monitor, and we look for any differences between the two sets of images, to find out whether there have been changes in any of the moles. This approach is reserved for special circumstances.

Total-body exam, dermoscopy, total-body photographs, and short-term monitoring provide a very powerful combination of tools for detecting melanomas. One significant advantage of such careful monitoring is that it reduces unnecessary biopsies of benign (normal) lesions. The efficacy of this system of approaches has been studied well in Europe, Australia, and the United States. A large number of scientific studies have been published to demonstrate its benefits. Let me emphasize that this approach does not replace skin biopsies, however. Instead, this system helps to increase diagnostic accuracy and works especially well for high-risk melanoma patients.

Perform Regular Self-Exams of Your Skin

Routinely examining your skin is crucial. People who have a personal history of melanoma have a higher risk of developing subsequent melanomas and other skin cancers than do people in the general population. The risk of developing new lesions or of having the original tumor come back is especially high in the first five years after the initial melanoma diagnosis. That is why patients need to perform skin exams on themselves once a month, *every month.*

A significant proportion of all melanomas are brought to the physicians' attention by the patients themselves. Some studies have estimated that nearly 75 percent of new melanomas are found by patients, their friends, or their family members.

Patients often ask, "What should I look for?" or "What are the clues of melanoma?" They want to perform self-examinations, but they have no idea what they should be looking for. Physicians can sympathize with their concern, because accurate diagnosis of melanoma is not easy. It is difficult even for dermatologists. You can improve your ability to spot worrisome lesions by following these strategies.

Use the ABCDE rule. This memory aid was created by melanoma specialists at New York University more than twenty years ago. The purpose of their project was to highlight the specific features of melanomas visible to the naked eye, and in this way to help phy-

Table 3.4. How to Perform a Skin Self-Examination

Step 1. Select a private, comfortable, and well-lit place. Use a mirror to look at areas such as your back and the back of your legs.

Step 2. Examine your entire body. Make sure you look at the bottoms of your feet and at your scalp. Melanomas in these two areas carry a poor prognosis; you want to find them early.

Step 3. Develop a systematic approach in your exam, checking body parts in the same sequence each time. Here is my recommended routine. Start by looking at your left hand and arm, and then switch over to the right arm and hand. Then examine your chest and abdomen, and turn around to look over your back. This is followed by checking your legs and feet. Lastly, examine your face and scalp. Consider recording the locations of all the moles or lesions on a body map—an outline of your body—front and back. In addition to the location, also write down the size of the lesions. You may even want to take some digital photos of any worrisome lesions for comparison at a later time.

Step 4. Ask for help. Have a family member or a good friend look over your back and other hard-to-see areas. If you are alone, use two mirrors, a full-length mirror and a hand-held mirror, for help.

sicians and the public to spot this deadly skin cancer at an early stage. Initially, the "E" was not included, but now "E" is considered to be an important feature as well. Table 3.5 spells out the system and Figure 3.2 gives some examples.

Look for the "ugly duckling" sign. This term refers to a lesion on the skin that does not share the same appearance as the moles in the nearby surrounding skin (see Figure 3.3). During a self-exam, first scan an entire anatomic region as a whole, looking for any feature that stands out. For example, quickly scan your entire back or entire chest and pay attention to any moles that stand out from their neighboring moles. A particular mole may be darker in color, asymmetrical in shape, or just larger in size. This mole is called the "ugly duckling" because it looks different from its neighbors.

Pay attention to symptoms. Pay special attention to any moles or lesions that are painful, itching, or bleeding and any that have

Table 3.5. The ABCDE Guidelines for Monitoring Lesions

A stands for *a*symmetry of the lesion. This focuses on the shape of a lesion. If a lesion could fold on itself in two directions without overlap, it is said to be symmetrical in two axes. In general, *a*symmetrical lesions are worrisome.

B stands for *b*order irregularities. In general, lesions with irregular (not smooth) borders are worrisome.

C stands for multiple *c*olors. In general, lesions with many colors are a cause for concern.

D stands for *d*iameter of the lesion greater than 6 mm, which is about the size of a pencil head eraser.

E stands for *e*volution, or change in shape, color, size, or symptoms.

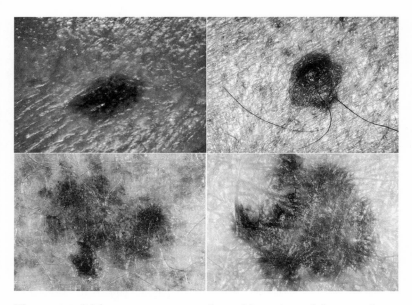

Figure 3.2. Melanomas can appear in a wide variety of shapes, colors, forms, and sizes—many more than can be illustrated by photographs. For more examples of melanoma see Figures C.1–C.5 in the color illustrations. Each of these four photos shows the ABCD features of melanomas (see Table 3.5). Color versions of these photographs follow Figure C.5, immediately preceding the glossary.

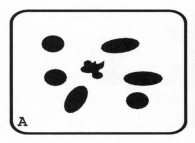 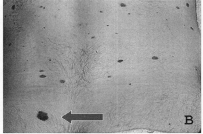

Figure 3.3. The "ugly duckling sign" refers to a lesion that looks different from its neighbors. (A) Drawn illustration. (B) Photograph of a large atypical lesion (arrow) that looks different from its neighboring moles.

changed in shape, color, or size since you last examined your skin. See your doctor and show him or her these moles or lesions and describe the symptoms carefully. If you have kept a body map and/ or notes during your skin self-exams (see Table 3.4), bring those along when you see your physicians.

These three strategies—the ABCDE rule, the ugly duckling sign, and paying attention to symptoms—work well for detecting worrisome lesions. Do not be concerned if, when you first start performing these scheduled self-exams, you find it difficult. Many of my patients tell me that they do not know if they are doing the exam correctly, and some patients stop doing their skin exams because they have so many doubts about what they are seeing or they become anxious about every little spot. Your main goal in performing self-exams is not to train yourself to diagnose skin cancers. You are not expected to achieve a high diagnostic accuracy in spotting early melanomas. If that is your goal, you should become a dermatologist.

Instead, the main goal of skin self-examination is for you and anyone who helps you to become familiar with your moles and lesions. You are looking for changes and symptoms. You are providing another pair of eyes to help your doctor spot worrisome lesions. If you find some moles or lesions that are of concern to you, you should consult your physicians. Over time you will get better at distinguishing benign lesions from worrisome ones. I know vigilant high-risk patients who have become rather good at spotting worrisome lesions over the years.

In addition to helping detect melanomas early, another benefit of the self skin exam is that a routine self-exam will help you practice other behaviors that can prevent skin cancers. Doing these monthly exams will remind you to avoid excessive UV exposure, wear protective clothing, and wear sunscreen on a daily basis. The goal is long-term, consistent behavior modification, much like the way maintaining an exercise regimen helps people watch their diet. The act of daily exercise helps to remind and motivate individuals to follow an overall healthy lifestyle.

Why You Should Not Use Tanning Booths

Nearly everyone reading this book will have heard about the potential harms associated with tanning booths. This issue is so important, however, that I am going to weigh in on it, too.

The tanning industry is a billion-dollar business. Thousands of tanning salons have sprouted up across cities and suburbs in the United States. Tanning franchises market their services by tapping into our society's misguided notion that tanned skin is attractive and sexy. They promote the idea that tanned skin conveys an impression of wealth and affluence.

The industry also tells potential customers about supposed benefits of using artificial tanning booths. However, most of these so-called health benefits are false. For instance, tanning salons often tell their customers that a tan will help to prevent sunburn. This message is very appealing to individuals planning vacations in sunny climates, but the truth is that the tan generated by artificial tanning provides a paltry SPF of 2 to 3. More importantly, current science tells us that a tan is the body's response to biological damages on a cellular level.

The tanning industry also promotes the notion that tanning increases vitamin D synthesis. However, the light sources in a tanning booth mainly emit UVA light, and UVB are the rays needed in vitamin D synthesis.

Artificial tanning is associated with the development of melanomas and also with the development of other skin cancers. Tanning also accelerates the aging process. About a year ago, one of my dermatologist colleagues consulted me on a case involving a 24-year-old man. The patient walked into my colleague's office and complained about diffuse reddish patches on his lower back. He confessed that he frequently visited a tanning salon. As my colleague examined those patches, he was perplexed initially. The diffuse and extensive nature of the rash was suggestive of psoriasis, but it was not typical psoriasis. As he looked closer, he noted blood vessels in some of these patches. He performed a biopsy on one of the patches. The result was rather surprising. It was a basal cell carcinoma, a common type of skin cancer. He then biopsied a few more patches; they were all basal cell carcinomas. This was a difficult case to manage. What should he do? What was the best way to treat these large areas of skin cancers on the back of a young man? Multiple surgeries would be needed to remove all of the cancers, and these procedures would leave many scars. After a lengthy discussion, my colleague decided to start a topical treatment as a trial. Most of the skin cancers were successfully treated with this topical medication, but the young man still needed surgeries to remove the lesions that did not respond to topical treatment. This story is an exceptional one, but it does highlight one of the potential health hazards associated with artificial tanning.

In my opinion, no one should use a tanning booth. Anyone who has a personal history of melanomas or other skin cancers *must not* use a tanning booth. If you have had any form of skin cancer, you should also tell your children and siblings to avoid tanning booths.

Medical Developments

Computer-Assisted Diagnostic Devices

To improve the accuracy of diagnoses of melanoma, research groups around the world have been engaged in developing equipment and analysis software that can detect melanoma. For many of these researchers, the ultimate objective is to develop a fully automated

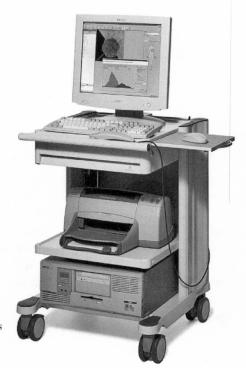

Figure 3.4. Dermogenius is an example of a computer-assisted diagnostic device.

diagnostic instrument with the capability of diagnosing skin cancers without the assistance of physicians.

These computer image and analysis systems all have many components. The image acquisition component captures and stores the image of the lesion. The image segmentation component automatically outlines the boundary between the lesion and the surrounding skin, visually separating the lesion from its surrounding normal skin. The analysis system looks over the image of the lesion only, and quantifies all the features of the lesion. In most systems, a score is generated. Depending on the score, a choice is made about whether the lesion in question is malignant.

A few of these systems have been incorporated into the clinical arena. Figure 3.4 is a picture of one example of an automated diagnostic system, the Dermogenius computer analysis system.

Some of these systems show a great deal of promise. However, so far, there is no automated system that is better than experienced specialists in the field.

MoleSafe

MoleSafe (www.molesafe.com) is a computerized melanoma screening program that aims to detect melanoma at the earliest possible stage. The program was started in New Zealand and then spread to Australia (in both countries, the incidence of melanoma is very high). The founder of this program understood that early detection is the key to a good outcome. In 2008, the program was launched in the United States, from headquarters in New Jersey. Molesafe currently provides this service in only a few centers in the United States.

The program starts by compiling a personal profile of the patient. Then, three types of digital images of the individual are taken by trained nurses or other health care staff. The first type of image is the total-body photograph, to capture all the moles or lesions on the body. The next two sets of images are close-up and dermoscopic images of any lesions that deserve attention. These images are stored in an encrypted software system.

All of the images and associated data are sent via a secure network to be reviewed by a panel of dermatologists and dermoscopists. They provide diagnoses and reports for each of the imaged lesions. The reports are sent to the patient and the patient's referring physician. Depending on the diagnosis, the patient may be prompted to have certain lesions removed or may be instructed to have regular follow-up. Patients also receive a CD of the clinical images.

Confocal Laser Microscopy

A confocal laser microscope is an imaging device designed to examine skin tissue in a noninvasive fashion (see Figure 3.5). Like x-ray, MRI, and CT imaging used to see internal organs, the confocal laser microscope delivers high-resolution images of skin, showing rich detail of individual skin cells and their nuclei. The technology is so amazing that it can even picture individual red blood cells tumbling through the blood vessels.

The clarity and magnification of confocal laser microscopy are comparable to those of standard microscopes. However, while a biopsy is required before tissue can be examined under a standard microscope, skin tissue can be examined under confocal laser microscopy without a biopsy of the skin tissue. Aside from the noninvasive nature and high-resolution imaging of the device, a confocal laser microscope can also examine the skin tissue layer by layer. By adjusting the focus plane in the device, the physician can selectively look at the layer of skin that is of interest.

Confocal laser microscopy has been refined and improved since it was first introduced into the clinical setting as a research tool in the 1980s. It has transitioned from a tool used purely for research purposes into a tool used in patient care. One of its clinical applications is to diagnose and treat melanomas. Specialists and researchers around the world have used confocal laser microscopy to improve their diagnostic accuracy of melanoma. The device is especially useful for detecting lentigo melanoma, a type of melanoma commonly found on the face. Using this device, the physicians can decide whether a lesion on the face needs a biopsy or not. More important, the device can guide the physicians in deciding exactly where to biopsy. For some physicians, the ultimate goal is to use the device to map out the border of melanomas on the face before performing the definitive surgery, so that as little skin tissue as possible need be removed.

Currently, the device is used by only a handful of dermatological centers around the country, and only a small number of specialists have the training and knowledge to use the device effectively. These specialist researchers and physicians hope to refine the technology even further and teach other clinicians how to use this tool.

Genetic Analysis

A new technology being developed by Dermtech, Inc., also aims to increase the accuracy of melanoma diagnoses, but it takes a

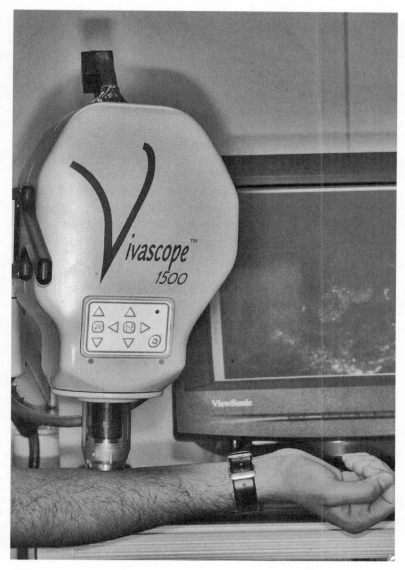

Figure 3.5. A confocal laser microscope.

completely different approach from some of the other medical advances. Instead of using enhanced imaging to assist diagnosis, it uses the genetic information in the cells. Special tape is used to remove cells on the very top layer of the skin at the site of a lesion of interest. The materials harvested with the tape are processed to extract the genetic content. Based on the genetic information, a data analysis system determines whether the lesion is a melanoma or a benign mole.

The major benefit of this technique is that no invasive biopsy is needed. Currently, the analysis system uses selected genes to separate melanomas from normal skin and benign moles. In a small study with a small number of melanomas and benign moles, the tape stripping analysis system demonstrated the feasibility of making the correct diagnosis at a high level of accuracy. This technology is promising, but much more work is needed to confirm the preliminary results.

4. Networking

Finding and Sharing Information

As a person with melanoma, you have read in this book about the importance of identifying melanoma early, getting good treatment from specialists with expertise, and taking steps to prevent melanoma. What else might you do? I would strongly urge you to network with other people who have had melanoma. By sharing your story with others, you may help some people avoid melanoma and help other people cope with melanoma and get good treatment. Helping others will also make you feel better. And, in telling your story, you will have a chance to think through your experience and continue to come to terms with it.

One way to network with other people concerned about melanoma is to get involved with the melanoma support groups and nonprofit organizations that have been established to help people with melanoma. These organizations will help you to learn more about the nature of the disease and to keep up with the advances being made in care for individuals with melanomas. The accumulation of knowledge will reduce your anxiety and concerns and will aid you in leading a healthy lifestyle that will reduce your risk of developing additional skin cancers.

After beating melanoma, you will have walked through a difficult journey. You may remember the roller coaster of emotions and thoughts you had during the "mad rush" phase. You have knowledge and personal experience that can be helpful to many other individuals with newly diagnosed melanoma. Although physicians play the major roles in patient care, you, too, can help. By sharing your experience and offering advice to others, you will provide assistance to many in a moment of need. Many individuals with newly diagnosed melanomas will want to hear your perspective and hear about your experience. You are not only another patient; you are a melanoma survivor! In addition, the process of sharing your stories and experience can be very cathartic for you. Support groups provide a channel through which many of my own patients release their own concerns and anxieties.

How Can I Get Involved?

Keep learning. Visit the Web sites listed below and in Chapter 2. These Web sites provide reliable information about cancer.

Keep up to date about products that reduce UV exposure. Remember, UV exposure is the most significant cause of melanoma and other skin cancers. In the next few years, we will see many innovative and improved products come to the market. Some of the Web sites listed below will carry information about these products. Visit www.skincancer.org and www.melanomapictures.org.

Donate. A number of nonprofit organizations in this country were created to fight melanomas and skin cancers. Some of these organizations are listed below. Your donation does not have to be in the form of a monetary contribution, although money is the easiest commodity to donate. You can get involved with these or-ganizations in several other ways, too: you can donate your time, expertise, connections, and skills. All these forms of assistance will be appreciated. For example, one of my patients is a marketing director for a large wine distribution company in New Jersey. He hosts an annual wine tasting event the proceeds from which are donated to the Melanoma Foundation. One teenage patient created cartoon illustrations for a nonprofit company that uses the pictures to teach children about the importance of protecting oneself from excessive sun exposure.

Recommended Web Sites

American Academy of
Dermatology
847-240-1280
www.aad.org

American Melanoma Foundation
619-448-0991
www.melanomafoundation.org

American Cancer Society
800-ACS-2345
www.cancer.org

Melanoma International
Foundation
866-463-6663
www.melanomaintl.org

National Cancer Institute
800-4-CANCER
www.nci.nih.gov

Shade Foundation
866-417-4233
www.shadefoundation.org

The Skin Cancer Foundation
212-725-5176
www.skincancer.org

The Wellness Community
202-659-9709
www.thewellnesscommunity.org

www.MelanomaPictures.org

Chapter 5. Beating Melanoma
The Checklist

The first part of this book provided a step-by-step guide to beating melanoma. The second part of the book described how to avoid developing melanoma and how to find additional information. This short chapter brings the two parts of the book together in an at-a-glance checklist. Even without the stress of a melanoma diagnosis, it is easy to forget or lose track of tasks when we all have so many things to do. This list will, I hope, make it easier for you to work your way through the important steps in melanoma treatment and prevention.

1. "Mad Rush" Phase

- ☐ Obtain a physical copy of your pathology report.
- ☐ Read and understand the report.
  - ☐ Where is my melanoma located?
  - ☐ Is it in situ or invasive?
  - ☐ What is the Breslow thickness?
  - ☐ Is ulceration or mitosis present?
- ☐ Assess the reliability of the report. Do you and your physicians feel confident about the diagnosis?
- ☐ Find the experts in your area.
- ☐ Determine the stage of your disease by asking your doctor or by reading the AJCC staging system guidelines and calculating it yourself.
- ☐ Understand the treatment options. Discuss all the options with your doctors.
- ☐ Understand the possible outcomes. Discuss your prognosis with your doctors.

2. "Marathon" Phase

- ☐ Are you routinely seeing a dermatologist?
- ☐ Are you routinely seeing an oncologist or a surgeon, if needed?
- ☐ How frequently are you being followed by these doctors? Ask your doctor what he or she recommends in terms of follow-up schedule, and keep to the schedule.
- ☐ Determine your risk factors for developing additional melanomas.
- ☐ Are you practicing monthly self-exam of your skin?
- ☐ Are you preventing excessive UV exposure?
  - ☐ Do you wear protective clothing and hats?
  - ☐ Do you use shade to protect yourself?
  - ☐ Do you use sunscreens?

Appendix A

Basal Cell Cancer

Every year, more than one million new cases of skin cancer are diagnosed in the United States. The most common type of skin cancer is basal cell cancer, which accounts for 80 percent of all diagnosed skin cancers. Basel cell cancers can grow and destroy local surrounding tissue, especially if they are left untreated for a long time. Fortunately, basal cell cancer rarely spreads to other parts of the body.

Basal cell cancer, like other skin cancer, is caused mainly by excessive ultraviolet radiation exposure. People with fair skin or who sunburn easily are at greatest risk for developing this cancer. Other potential risks for developing this cancer include a history of x-ray radiation, arsenic exposure, a major thermal burn, and a chronic wound that does not heal.

Most basal cell cancers are found on sun-exposed sites, such as the head, forehead, eyelids, nose, ears, neck and back. There are many variants of basal cell cancer, with a wide range of presentations ("presentation" is doctor-talk for how they look and act).

A common type of basal cell cancer is the *nodular type*. It presents as a small pink or red nodule with a translucent appearance. Upon close inspection, small blood vessels may be visible. As the nodule grows, the center may become ulcerated.

Another very common variant is the *superficial type*. Typically, it is a flat lesion that is pink or red in color. A small amount of scale may be seen on it.

Another type of basal cell cancer is the *morpheaform type*. Typically, this type has a raised texture and is an ivory color. Blood vessels may be seen in it.

Some basal cell cancers have dark pigmentation or colors. Those are the *pigmented type*. Very often, this variant can look like melanoma.

Treatment for basal cell cancer includes the following:

Mohs surgery
radiation
topical medications, such as Aldara
cryotherapy
electrodessication and curettage
standard excision
photodynamic therapy

For more information about these treatments, talk with your doctor. Many of the organizations recommended in Chapter 4 can provide additional information about basal cell cancers and their treatment.

Examples of basal cell cancers are shown in Figures A.1–A.7 in the color illustrations. Basal cell cancers may have many other appearances beyond those illustrated here.

Appendix B

Squamous Cell Cancer

Of the more than one million new cases of skin cancer diagnosed in the United States each year, about 15 percent are squamous cell cancers, the second most common type of skin cancer. For most squamous cell cancers, the treatment is relatively straightforward and the cure rate is excellent. However, there is a subset of squamous cell cancers that are rather aggressive. They can cause extensive local tissue destruction and may recur after treatment. Some of these squamous cell cancers have the potential to spread to other distant parts of the body and even lead to death.

As with other types of skin cancer, the cause of squamous cell cancer can be attributed to both environmental exposure and genetic predisposition. People with fair skin who sunburn easily are at greatest risk for developing this cancer. Ultraviolet radiation from the sun or other sources is the major culprit causing this skin cancer. More than 80 percent of all squamous cell cancers are found on sun-exposed surfaces such as the head, neck, and upper extremities. People who have received a transplanted organ are at an extremely high risk for developing this type of skin cancer because of the immunosuppressive drugs they must take. Other environmental exposure factors include soot, pitch and tar, shale oil, and arsenic.

The presentation of squamous cell cancer varies considerably ("presentation" means how they look and act). In general, most squamous cell cancers develop in the background of sun-damaged skin. Most squamous cell cancer patients have actinic keratosis, a type of precancerous spot that is red in color, has scales and is rough to the touch. Most early squamous cell cancers have a rough scale. As the tumors grow, they enlarge into a nodule with or without ulceration. Large tumors can also produce pain, can ulcerate, and can weep blood or other fluid.

Treatments for squamous cell cancer include the following:

Mohs surgery
radiation
topical medication, such as Aldara and Carac
cryotherapy
electrodessication and curettage
standard excision
photodynamic therapy

For more information about these treatments, talk with your doctor. Many of the organizations recommended in Chapter 4 can provide additional information about squamous cell cancers and their treatment.

Examples of squamous cell cancers are shown in Figures B.1– B.5 in the color illustrations. Squamous cell cancers may have many other appearances beyond those illustrated here.

Appendix C
Melanoma Image Library

Examples of melanoma are shown in Figures C.1–C.5 in the color illustrations. Melanoma may have many other appearances beyond those illustrated here. If you have a lesion that looks like one of these pictures, *you may have melanoma or you may have another type of skin cancer, or you may not have a skin cancer at all.*

If you are worried about any spots, lesions, or moles on your body, you need to consult a qualified medical professional without delay.

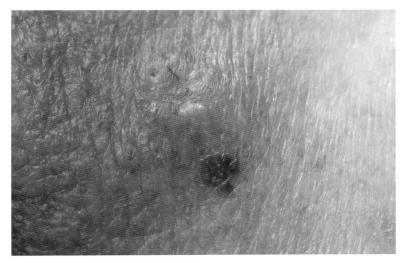

A.1

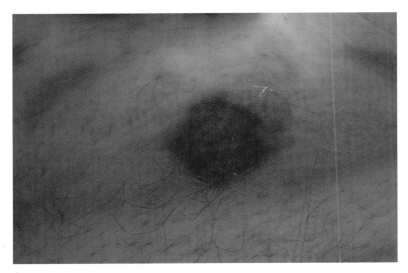

A.2

Examples of basal cell cancers

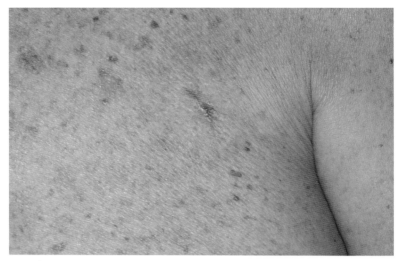

A.3

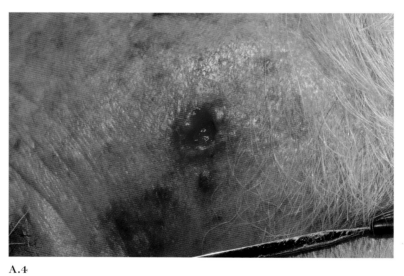

A.4

Examples of basal cell cancers

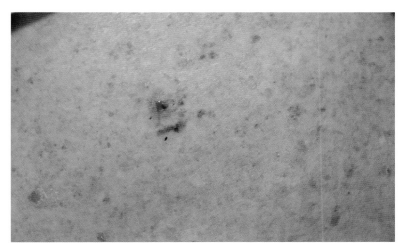

A.5

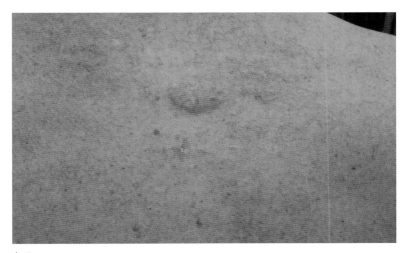

A.6

Examples of basal cell cancers

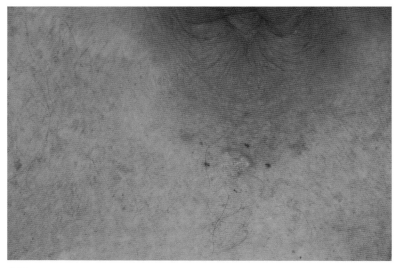

A.7

Example of basal cell cancer

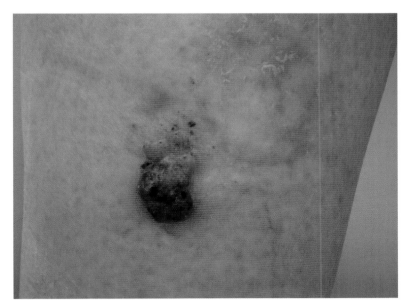

B.1

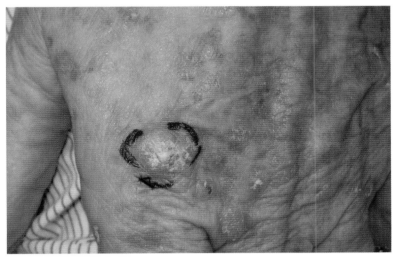

B.2

Examples of squamous cell cancers

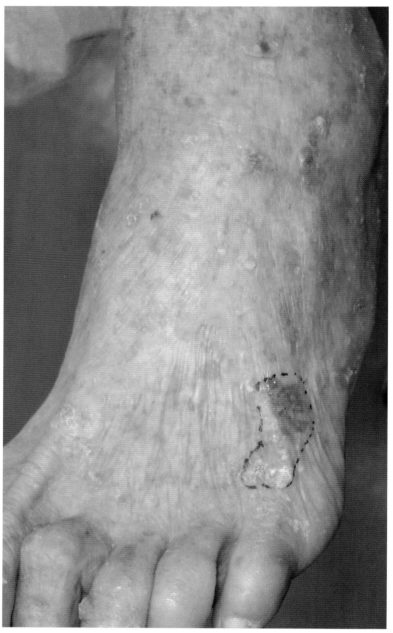

B.3

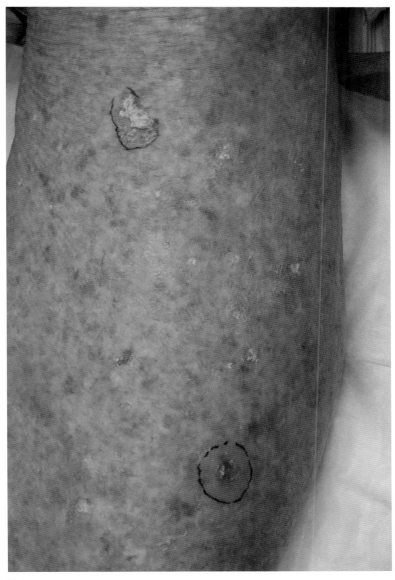

B.4

Examples of squamous cell cancers *here and facing*

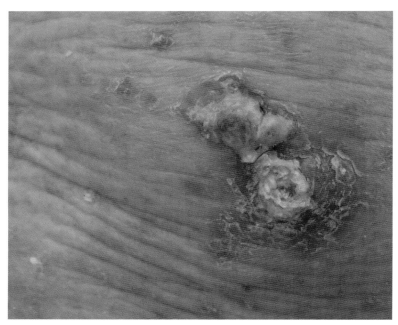

B.5

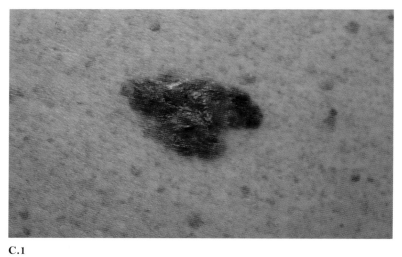

C.1

Squamous cell cancer *top*, melanoma *bottom*

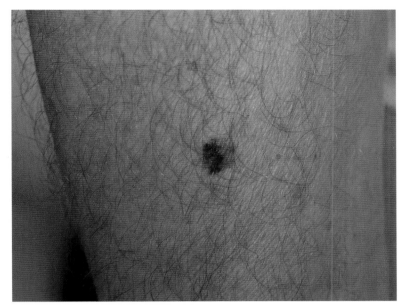

C.2

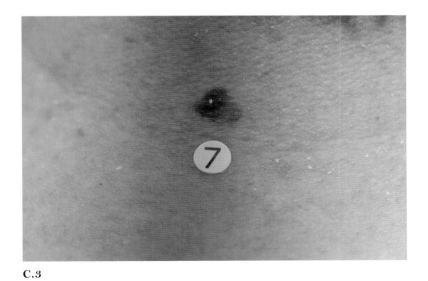

C.3

Examples of melanomas

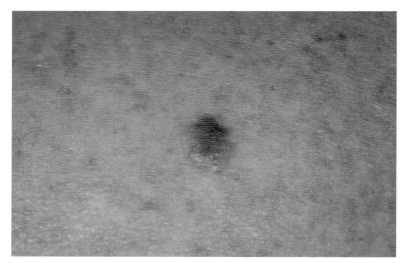

C.4

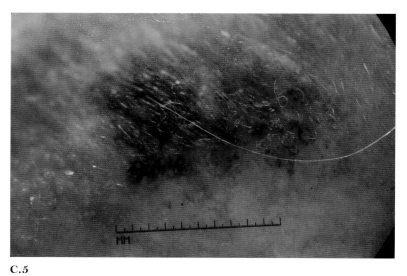

C.5

Examples of melanomas

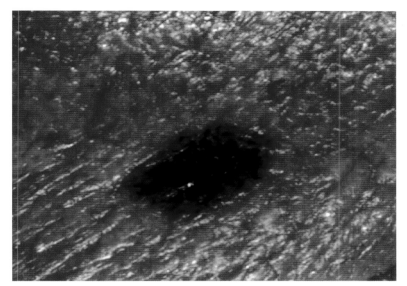

3.2A

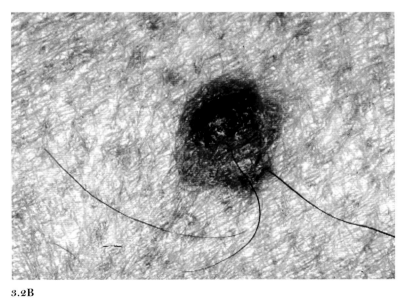

3.2B

Chapter 3 figures

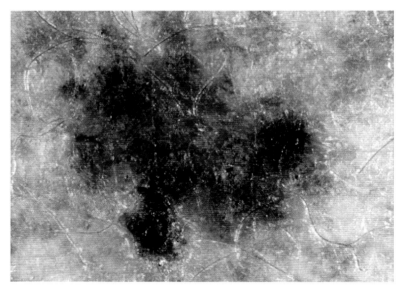

3.2C

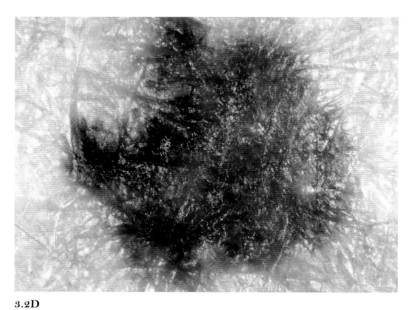

3.2D

Chapter 3 figures

Glossary

ABCDE. Abbreviation used to help the public and health care providers identify and remember clinical features of melanoma (see Table 3.5).

actinic keratosis. A type of precancerous skin spot that is red in color, has scales, and is rough to the touch.

adjuvant therapy. Secondary treatment delivered to enhance the effectiveness of the primary treatment and help prevent recurrence of the disease.

alpha interferon. A type of immunotherapy that aims to boost the body's immune system. Used to treat several diseases, including cancer.

atypical nevi. Moles that resemble melanoma in appearance. Another name for these moles is dysplastic nevi.

basal cell carcinoma. The most common type of skin cancer.

benign. Normal. Not cancerous.

biopsy. Taking a small piece of skin tissue for diagnosis by microscopic examination.

blood count. The number of red cells, white cells, and platelets in a blood sample.

board certified. Physicians who have completed a requirement specified by their specialty board.

Breslow thickness. Measurement of the depth of penetration by the tumor cells, taken from the very top of the epidermis (outermost layer of the skin) to the deepest melanoma cells in the skin tissue.

cancer. A class of illnesses characterized by the proliferation of cells that invade and destroy normal surrounding tissue and have the potential to spread throughout the body.

CBC. Complete blood count. Measures the number of white blood cells (WBCs), red blood cells, and platelets.

cell. The basic unit of living organism.

centimeter (cm). A hundredth of a meter; about 4 tenths of an inch.

chemotherapy. Treatment with a class of drugs used to destroy cancer.

Clark level. A common way for pathologists to report the depth of melanoma invasion.

clinical trial. Medical study evaluating the efficacy of experimental drugs for treating cancer or other diseases.

confocal laser microscopy. An imaging method designed to examine the cellular structures within skin tissue in a noninvasive fashion.

congenital mole. A mole that is found at birth. The size of a congenital mole can vary from a few millimeters to larger than 20 centimeters.

cryotherapy. Treatment that freezes benign or malignant skin lesions with liquid nitrogen.

CT scan. Computed tomography scan. A series of x-ray views of the body from different angles. The images are combined and reconstructed by computer and reviewed by a radiologist. Sometimes called a CAT (computerized axial tomography) scan.

cure rate. The percentage of patients with a disease who have been cured, as determined by statistical studies.

curettage. A method of treating skin cancer by scraping away the tumor cells.

dermatologist. A physician who specializes in diagnosing and treating skin problems.

dermis. The lower layer of the skin found immediately below the epidermis (outermost) layer.

dermoscope. A hand-held microscope-like device that allows physicians to see deeper layers of the skin in a noninvasive fashion.

DNA (deoxyribonucleic acid). Nucleic acid contains the genetic information of living organisms.

dysplastic nevi. See **atypical nevi.**

electrodessication. A method of treating benign or malignant skin lesions using high-energy electrical currents or heat.

epidermis. The outermost or uppermost layer of the skin, located above the dermis layer.

excisional biopsy. A surgical procedure in which a piece of tumor or skin tissue is removed. The specimen is examined under a microscope for diagnosis.

Food and Drug Administration (FDA). A division of the federal government that regulates the safety and efficacy of drugs.

freckles. Light brown pigmentations found on the skin.

gene. A strand of DNA molecules needed by cells to produce and encode proteins.

gene therapy. Treatment that targets gene mutations.

groin. The area of the body where the thigh meets the hip and abdomen.

high-risk melanoma. Aggressive or advanced stage of melanoma that has a high probability of coming back, or recurring.

immune system. The body's defensive mechanism for combatting illness. It is an elaborate system composed of different types of immune cells that work together to identify, seek, and destroy viruses, bacteria, and cancer cells.

immunosuppression. A condition, caused by illness or certain therapies, in which the effectiveness of a person's immune system is reduced.

in situ. Latin for "in place," in this case meaning "in the original place." Used in reference to a skin cancer that is restricted to the epidermis, the first layer of the skin.

interferons. Proteins produced by white blood cells that boost the effectiveness of specific immune cells.

Interleukin-2 (IL-2). A molecule that boosts the body's innate immune cells. It is approved by the FDA for treating melanoma.

intravenous (IV). Into a vein. Usually describes medicine being delivered through the bloodstream.

isolated limb perfusion. A medical procedure in which a tourniquet is placed around an arm or a leg to cut off blood circulation from the rest of the body. High-dose chemotherapeutic drugs are then infused into the isolated limb. The purpose of this procedure is to deliver high doses of drugs to the local site of a cancer without causing significant damage to other parts of the body.

lesion. Abnormal tissue found on or in the body. It can be either benign or malignant.

lymphedema. Swelling of the arm or leg due to an accumulation of excess lymphatic fluid. The condition commonly occurs in patients who have had surgical procedures to remove lymph vessels or lymph nodes.

lymph nodes. Small bean-shaped immunologic structures (*see* immune system) connected to the lymphatic vessels, which are found throughout the body. They contain various immunologic cells (for example, T and B cells) and can become enlarged or painful when the body is fighting illnesses ranging from infection to cancers.

malignant. Cancerous. Malignant tumors or cells can destroy nearby normal tissue and can spread to other parts of the body.

melanocytes. Specialized pigment-producing cells located in the bottom layer of the epidermis. Melanoma is derived from cancerous melanocytes.

melanoma. A type of skin cancer derived from cancerous melanocytes.

metastasis. The spread of cancer cells from one part of the body to another part of the body via the bloodstream or the lymphatic system.

metastatic melanoma. Melanoma that has spread from the original site to other parts of the body, such as the bone, brain, liver or other parts of the skin.

mitosis. The multiplication of cells by division, the splitting of one cell into two cells.

mole. A collection of melanocytes in the skin. A mole appears as a brown, black, or flesh-colored spot on the skin. Also called a nevus.

MRI. Magnetic resonance imaging, a medical imaging technique used to visualize internal structures of the body.

nevus (plural, **nevi**). *See* mole.

nodule. A type of growth found in the body.

oncologist. A physician who specializes in treating cancer.

pathologist. A physician who specializes in diagnosing diseases by examining tissues and cells under the microscope.

PET scan. Positron emission tomography. A nuclear imaging technology capable of detecting areas of the body that contain malignant cells.

photodynamic therapy. A method of treating benign or malignant skin lesions using a combination of light and chemicals.

plastic surgeon. A surgeon who specializes in restoring function and normal appearance to parts of the body altered by disease or by surgery (such as removal of cancerous lesions).

prognosis. A prediction of the probable outcome of a disease.

radiation oncologist. A physician who specializes in radiation treatment for cancer.

recurrence. The reappearance of a cancer or disease after a period of remission.

remission. Disappearance of a cancer or chronic illness.

resection. Surgical removal of tissue, such as a malignant tumor.

RNA. Ribonucleic acid is produced from DNA and is important in protein production.

sentinel lymph node. The first lymph node or nodes which malignant tumor cells reach when cancer spreads from its original site.

sentinel lymph node biopsy. A surgical procedure to remove and examine the sentinel lymph node to determine if cancerous cells are present.

side effects. Secondary effects, sometimes harmful, of a drug or therapy that may occur in addition to the primary effect.

SPF. Sun protection factor. A standard for measuring the efficacy of sunscreen in protecting against (mainly) the UVB portion of solar radiation.

squamous cell carcinoma. A type of skin cancer.

sunscreen. A substance applied to the skin to block or reflect ultraviolet radiation from the sun.

survival rate. The percentage of patients with a particular disease who have survived after treatment, as determined by statistical studies.

tumor. An abnormal growth of tissue. A tumor can be either benign (not cancerous) or malignant (cancerous).

ulceration. Open area on the skin or in tissue where there is breakdown of the tissue.

ultrasound. An imaging procedure using sound waves to visualize soft tissue and body cavities.

ultraviolet (UV) radiation. A spectrum of invisible rays from the sun or a sun lamp. UV radiation can cause skin cancer and can accelerate aging.

vaccine. An inactivated disease agent or biological substance given to create or improve immunity for a specific disease.

vitamin D. A fat soluble vitamin that helps strengthen bones and can be obtained from sun exposure, food sources, and vitamin supplements.

Index

About the Author

Steven Q. Wang, M.D., is the Director of Dermatologic Surgery and Dermatology at the Memorial Sloan-Kettering Cancer Center at Basking Ridge, New Jersey. He serves on the Photobiology Committee of the Skin Cancer Foundation. Dr. Wang specializes in the diagnosis, treatment, and prevention of skin cancers, especially melanoma. In the management of high-risk skin cancer patients, he uses whole-body photography, dermoscopy, and computerized digital imaging systems. In addition, he is actively involved in clinical research, with a focus on photoprotection and noninvasive imaging technologies to diagnose skin cancer. He is the author of more than fifty publications in peer-reviewed medical journals and academic textbooks. He has lectured extensively in the United States and around the world on the diagnosis, treatment, and prevention of melanoma and nonmelanoma skin cancers.

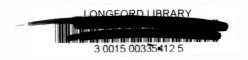